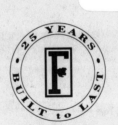

D0450462

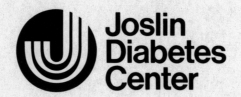

THE
JOSLIN
GUIDE TO DIABETES
A program for managing your treatment

RICHARD S. BEASER, M.D.,

with Joan V.C. Hill, R.D., C.D.E.,
and the Joslin Education Committee

A FIRESIDE BOOK

Published by Simon & Schuster
New York   London   Toronto   Sydney   Tokyo   Singapore

FIRESIDE
Rockefeller Center
1230 Avenue of the Americas
New York, NY 10020

Designed by Irving Perkins Associates

Manufactured in the United States of America

10

Library of Congress Cataloging-in-Publication Data

Beaser, Richard S.
    The Joslin guide to diabetes : a program for managing your
treatment / Richard S. Beaser, with Joan V. C. Hill and the Joslin
Education Committee.
        p.   cm.
    "A Fireside book".
    Includes index.
    1. Diabetes—Popular works.   I. Hill, Joan V. C.   II. Joslin
Diabetes Center. Joslin Education Committee.   III. Title.
RC660.4.B43   1995
616.4'62—dc20   95-12169
                                                          CIP

ISBN 0-684-80208-2

Information from the following titles was incorporated into this book with the permis-
sion of the Joslin Diabetes Center:
Fitting Alcohol into Your Meal Plan, 1994; *Joslin Diabetes Gourmet Cookbook,* 1994;
Eating Well, Living Better, 1992; *Good Health with Diabetes Through Exercise,* 1992;
Menu Planning, Simple, 1992; *Weight Loss: A Winning Battle,* 1992; *Diabetes Teach-
ing Guide for People Who Use Insulin,* 1989.

The authors gratefully acknowledge permission to use other copyrighted materials as
follows:
The Restaurant Companion, © 1995 Hope Warshaw, Surrey Books;
Outsmarting Diabetes, Richard Beaser, Chronimed Inc., 1994;
Joslin Diabetes Manual, 12th edition, © Lea & Febiger, 1989.

Contents

6   Contents

Introduction

IF YOU HAVE DIABETES, you have every reason to have confidence and hope. In recent years, medical science has made many advances that can help you lead a long, active, and productive life. However, you must take your condition seriously. Diabetes is a complex disease. Unlike many health problems that can be completely cured with the right treatment, there is no way to cure diabetes. It is a condition that you must deal with for the rest of your life. If you have diabetes, you will want to make sure that you have the best possible information in order to make the proper decisions about your health.

The statistics themselves are grim enough. Diabetes is the nation's third leading fatal disease, behind heart disease and cancer, annually killing an estimated 150,000 people in the United States and millions more throughout the world. Diabetes is the leading cause of blindness in working-age Americans, the single leading cause of end-stage kidney failure, the leading cause of lower-extremity amputations, and a leading risk factor for heart disease and strokes. Beyond the medical ramifications of diabetes is the financial impact. The disease costs Americans more than $92 billion per year in health-care expenditures and lost productivity. The emotional costs—to those with the disease, their families and friends—are immeasurable.

But there's good news. A 10-year nationwide study completed in 1993, called the Diabetes Control and Complications Trial or DCCT, demonstrated that people with one type of diabetes (Type I) were able to reduce their risk of developing serious long-term complications by 50 percent or more by keeping their blood sugar as close to normal as possible. Many clinicians and researchers believe the results of this study show that anyone with diabetes can cut the risks of developing complications by keeping the blood sugar in as normal a range as possible.

The Joslin Guide to Diabetes has been written to lessen the risk of your becoming one of diabetes' statistics. As you read this guide, you will learn how the body works—and what goes wrong in diabetes. You'll also learn what you can do to keep your body working as normally as possible.

The book is designed to be used as a reference tool for people with diabetes who are under the care of a physician and other health-care professionals. It was written by a team of experts in the field of diabetes care and education at the Joslin Diabetes Center in Boston, Massachusetts. Founded in 1898 by Dr. Elliott P. Joslin, a pioneer in diabetes research and care, the Joslin Diabetes Center is affiliated with Harvard Medical School and has treated more than 180,000 people with diabetes during the past century. It is one of the world's most renowned institutions in the field of diabetes care and research.

Basic Facts and Figures

WHAT IS DIABETES? Diabetes is a disorder in the way your body turns food into energy. The problem centers around a substance called *insulin* and how your body produces and uses it. Insulin helps turn the food you eat into energy.

Let's look at the whole process. When you digest a meal, food enters your bloodstream as sugars. One obvious source of sugar is table sugar. Foods such as bread or pasta also contain starch which breaks down in the body into sugars. Even foods such as meat and the margarine on your bread all contribute to the sugar in your blood. But if sugar simply flows around in your bloodstream, it's of no use to your body's cells. Something is needed to signal the cells to admit the sugar. That's where insulin comes into the picture. It is the "key" that unlocks the body's cells, letting the sugar in. Once the sugar moves from your bloodstream into your cells, the cells use it to get the energy they need to function normally.

Now let's look at the scene without the star performer, insulin. Without insulin, your cells are not able to use sugar normally, and as a result, they don't get enough energy. Also, the sugar "backs up" into the blood. The sugar level rises too high and stays too high most of the time. This condition is called diabetes.

TYPES OF DIABETES. There are two main types of diabetes—Type I and Type II—and the main difference between them depends on whether or not your body can still make insulin. People with Type I diabetes—also called *insulin-dependent* or in the old days "juvenile diabetes"—produce little or no insulin at all. If you have this type of diabetes, your body depends upon daily insulin injections. Without these injections, you will not survive.

By contrast, people with Type II diabetes—also called *non-insulin-dependent* diabetes—produce at least some insulin in their bodies. Their problem is that the insulin doesn't work properly, and therefore they are unable to utilize their sugar properly. They do not need daily insulin injections to survive. In many cases, they can manage their diabetes through proper nutrition and exercise. They may also take oral medications, or pills, to boost the amount of insulin their bodies produce or improve how their bodies use insulin. However, some people with Type II diabetes do need to take daily injections of insulin to maintain good health, adding to the small amount of natural insulin produced by their bodies. They may not need insulin to survive, but they do need it to stay healthy.

AN OLD DISEASE, BUT NEW REMEDIES. More than 120 million people throughout the world currently have diabetes. About 13 million are in the United States, which means that one out of every 20 people in this country has diabetes. The severity and the widespread nature of this condition have led scientists to do extensive research on diabetes, looking for ways to prevent and treat it. Their work all over the world has resulted in significant progress, particularly in the twentieth century. But medical descriptions of diabetes date back to at least 1500 B.C., nearly 3,500 years ago. Writings from ancient cultures in China and the Middle East describe the classic signs of diabetes, such as passing large quantities of urine through the body. The ancient Greeks gave us the name *diabetes*, which means "to flow through." Later, the Latin word *mellitus*, "sweetened or honeylike," was added to form the present medical name of *diabetes mellitus*.

Although diabetes has been known for thousands of years, the actual treatment of the disease was very basic. Until recent times, people with diabetes could use only diet, exercise, and weight control to try to treat their disorder. But then in 1921, a remarkable substance became available—insulin. The discovery of insulin was a major breakthrough in modern medicine, saving the lives of millions of people with diabetes. (In Part Three of this guide, you will learn about the possible use of insulin in your treatment program.) And research on diabetes continues to make major strides. New procedures are continually being developed to help people manage the disease. For example, you now can test your blood sugar by yourself—one of the most important advances in the care of diabetes since the discovery of insulin. Rather than depending solely on visits to the doctor to have your blood sugar tested, you can use a simple testing device to keep track of your blood sugar level on a regular basis, as often as several times each day if necessary. This means you can have better control of your diabetes, get more energy, and live a more flexible and free lifestyle.

Good diabetes control brings other benefits. By maintaining proper blood sugar levels, you can prevent or slow the progression of the long-term complications of the disease. These include problems with the eyes, nerves, kidneys, feet, skin, and cardiovascular system. By gaining increased control, you can reduce the risks of developing such complications.

Discovering You Have Diabetes

If you think back to the time just before you learned you had diabetes, you may remember having noticed changes in your health. If you have Type I, or insulin-dependent, diabetes, the unusual changes in your body may have included excessive thirst, frequent urination, unexplained weight loss, and constant hunger. You probably felt very tired and sluggish, due to the fact that your body was unable to properly convert food sugars into energy. You may also have had other physical problems, such as nausea, vomiting, abdominal pain, weakness, and rapid shallow breathing. Some people even experience a *diabetic coma*, a life-threatening condition caused by extremely high levels of ketones in the blood, substances that are produced by the body when it must rely solely on burning fat for energy.

If you have Type II, or non-insulin-dependent, diabetes, perhaps the news of your condition was totally unexpected. You may have learned that you have diabetes during a routine checkup or an unrelated visit to your doctor—without having experienced any noticeable symptoms of the disease. For example, tests performed on your blood during an annual physical may have detected high levels of sugar in your blood. Perhaps you felt tired for a period of time and visited your physician to determine the cause. If you are a woman, you may have suffered from frequent vaginal infections and sought help with those. Or maybe you sought medical help for an unexplained difficulty, such as blurred vision or an infection that was slow to heal.

However, some people with Type II diabetes discover their condition because they develop symptoms similar to those experienced by people with Type I diabetes. These symptoms include increased hunger, frequent urination, unusual thirst, and occasionally an unexplained weight loss. But because the symptoms are often so mild, the person has little reason to suspect anything is wrong.

Occasionally, Type II diabetes is diagnosed when people develop another illness, such as a bad case of the flu. Any illness is stressful for the body and may increase the level of sugar in the blood. People who already have undetected high levels of blood sugar may show a sudden increase to excessively high levels. They may experience many of the symptoms described for Type I diabetes. Allowed to continue, this situation can lead to even more serious conditions, such as diabetic coma.

Assessing Your Feelings

No doubt, you felt some type of stress even before you discovered you had diabetes. The symptoms of the disease—such as thirst, frequent urination, and unexplained weight loss—can be very disturbing. After all, no one likes to see changes taking place in the body and not know the reason why. And once you found out you had diabetes—either Type I or II—the stresses associated with its symptoms probably didn't go away. They were simply exchanged for other stresses. Questions about your condition and your future were probably foremost in your mind. How did this happen? What causes diabetes? Can it be cured? How will it affect my daily life? Can I keep my job? What will it cost? What lies ahead?

Such questions are steps in the right direction. They mean you are concerned about your health. After all, you have a right to be concerned. Diabetes is a serious condition for which there is no known cure. Physicians are not even sure what causes diabetes or how to prevent it. However, research during the past decades has brought us closer to answering these vitally important questions. That's why, despite the seriousness of diabetes, there are many reasons to be hopeful.

However, managing your diabetes will not be easy and carefree. No one can promise you a completely normal life. There are things you must do to keep your condition under control. And there are things you must *not* do. In facing these issues, you may feel discouraged or frustrated at times. To place things in a proper perspective, you should make an honest assessment of your situation. That point exists somewhere between two extremes. Think of it as sitting too close or too far away from a fire. Each can be bad in its own way. You can make your problem "too hot" by worrying or becoming overly preoccupied with your diabetes; that is, trying to do too much. On the other hand, it's not good to be "too cold"—avoiding, denying, or minimizing your situation so that you don't take your care seriously. It's best to find a point in the middle, where your attitudes are comfortably "warm."

To help you with your feelings about diabetes, it's often a good idea to find someone in whom you can confide—perhaps your physician, a health-care professional, a family member, or a good friend. This person can be a valuable resource in helping you develop a healthy outlook about your condition.

Of equal importance, once you have been diagnosed with diabetes, is a complete understanding of its causes and methods of treatment. Diabetes is a uniquely personal condition and you are about to embark on a daily endeavor of self-care. In many ways, this is nothing new. Since birth, you've learned ways to take care of yourself—how to eat, dress for the weather, and protect yourself from harm. Now that you have diabetes, it may be helpful for you to think of your care as simply making an adjustment to these lifelong habits. In effect, you'll be changing certain parts of your lifestyle.

At first, you may ask yourself, "Can I really handle this?" Remember, your skills and confidence will grow as the weeks pass, and *The Joslin Guide to Diabetes* will help you develop that confidence. It will help you understand how your body works. It will show you how diabetes changes your body and how you can use nutrition, exercise, and medication to manage your condition. In addition to the care provided by your personal physician and health-care team, this guide will provide you with the knowledge and skills you need to care for your diabetes.

Diabetes is a complex condition. Understanding it and learning to care for yourself are ongoing, lifelong tasks. This guide, along with your physician and other health-care professionals, will help you learn what you need to know for your immediate and your long-term well-being. If you don't understand certain concepts or courses of treatment, do not hesitate to ask your physician or health-care team for help. They will be glad to assist you in your effort to care for your diabetes. Remember, the knowledge you have of this condition is much more than a *part* of the treatment—it *is* the treatment.

Part One

UNDERSTANDING DIABETES

CHAPTER 1

What Is Diabetes?

ANYTIME YOU WANT to learn about a medical problem, it's best to approach it in two steps. First, learn how the body functions normally. Then focus on what happens when something goes wrong. This is the best way to learn about diabetes, too. First, you need to understand how the body normally produces energy. You should then focus on how a breakdown in this process leads to the two major types of diabetes—either your body can't make any or enough insulin, or it can't properly use the insulin it produces.

How the Body Normally Produces Energy

Quite simply, you can't live without food. The body needs food to nourish itself and sustain life. Food is both "fuel" and "building material." It produces energy, builds and repairs body tissue, and regulates body functions. But before food is used by the cells, it's put through some biological paces. First, your body must break down the food you eat into its basic ingredients, or nutrients. These nutrients fall into three major categories—carbohydrates, proteins, and fats.

Carbohydrates are found in most foods. Often called "starches" and "sugars," they are found in bread, pasta, fruits, and vegetables. *Proteins* are found in meats, milk, and fish. *Fats* are found in such foods as vegetable oils, meat, cheese, and other dairy products. All these nutrients are digested, or broken down, in the stomach and intestines. Carbohydrates are broken down into a simple sugar called *glucose*, which passes through the wall of the intestines into your bloodstream. This is the form of sugar that is often called "blood glucose" or, more simply, just "blood sugar." Diabetes is a disorder in the way the body *uses* blood sugar, or glucose.

The Role of Insulin

Once glucose gets into your bloodstream, it circulates to the body's cells to provide them energy. But glucose can't simply flow into the cells. All cells are enclosed by a thin wall called a *membrane*, and something has to tell your cells that glucose is waiting outside. That something is insulin. It attaches on the outside of the cells to special sites called *insulin receptors*—much like a key that fits into a lock. Insulin is the "key" that unlocks the cells, allowing glucose to enter. Once inside, the glucose is metabolized, or "burned," by the cells for energy.

Exactly what kind of substance is insulin? It is a *hormone*—a chemical messenger made in one part of the body to transmit "information" through your bloodstream to cells in another part of the body. Your body produces many types of hormones. Insulin is a specific kind of hormone made in the organ called the *pancreas*.

The Pancreas

The pancreas is a small gland situated below and behind the stomach. In an adult, it weighs less than half a pound. The pancreas is shaped like a long cone lying on its side, with the end tapering off into a "tail." Within this tail are tiny bits of tissue called *islets of Langerhans*.

A normal pancreas has about 100,000 islets of Langerhans. But these islets are actually clusters of various types of cells. The most important are the *beta cells*—the tiny "factories" that make insulin. The beta cells also serve as "warehouses," storing insulin until it's needed by the body.

In addition to producing insulin, the pancreas has other important duties. Some cells produce hormones that are quite different from insulin, such as *glucagon*. This hormone actually *raises* the blood sugar—just the opposite function of insulin. The balancing act between insulin and glucagon helps keep blood sugar in the normal range, approximately 60–140 milligrams (mg) of sugar per deciliter (dl) of blood. Other cells in the pancreas produce substances called *enzymes*, which help in digestion by splitting foodstuffs into simpler substances, which can then be absorbed through the intestine into the bloodstream.

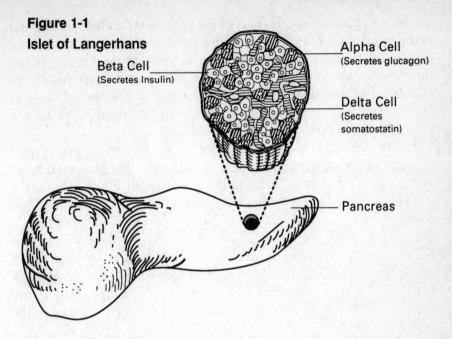

Figure 1-1
Islet of Langerhans

Beta Cell
(Secretes Insulin)

Alpha Cell
(Secretes glucagon)

Delta Cell
(Secretes somatostatin)

Pancreas

How Insulin Works

During normal digestion, enzymes in the stomach and intestines act upon the nutrients (carbohydrates, proteins, and fats), splitting them into simple substances, which enter the bloodstream in the following forms:

- Carbohydrates are converted into *glucose*, which is metabolized, or "burned," for energy.
- Proteins are converted into *amino acids*, which provide the basic building blocks for bone, muscle, and other tissues. Proteins also can be burned for energy.
- Fats become *fatty acids*, which are burned for energy or stored as body fat for later use. However, fat is burned differently from glucose, producing substances called *ketones*.

Insulin plays a role in the burning and storage of all these nutrients. In diabetes, however, its main role relates to the action of glucose, the simplified form of carbohydrates. The whole process works like a dietary drama. The key actors are the beta cells, which make and store insulin. When they sense the level of glucose rising in the blood, they respond by releasing just the right amount of insulin into the bloodstream.

At first, the beta cells release the insulin held in storage. But what if the body needs even more? This often happens right after a meal, and as the blood glucose levels increase, a second stage begins. The "control centers" of the beta cells trigger them to make more insulin. When functioning normally, the beta cells release just enough insulin to maintain the level of glucose in the blood within the normal range of 60–140 mg/dl, and once in the bloodstream, the insulin enables the glucose to enter your body's cells for energy.

Another process also occurs. Generally when you eat, you don't need to use all the glucose from your food immediately. The body takes some of the glucose and stores it for future needs. With insulin's help, the extra glucose is taken up by the liver cells and changed to a storage form called *glycogen*. Glycogen comes in handy when your body needs extra energy in a hurry, for instance, during exercise. At those times, your body rises to the occasion by quickly changing the stored glycogen back into glucose. In addition, this stored glucose takes care of your energy needs overnight, a time when you normally aren't eating. Insulin also helps convert some of the extra glucose into fat, which is stored in the body's fat cells.

What Goes Wrong in Diabetes?

Diabetes is caused by a breakdown in the normal processes described above. A breakdown can occur in one of two ways: (1) the body produces little or no insulin; or (2) the insulin that the body produces can't link up with the body's cells. Type I diabetes is the result of the first defect; Type II is the result of the second. It is important to note, however, that there are many similarities between Type I and Type II diabetes, and that some people display characteristics of both types.

Type I: Insulin-Dependent Diabetes

Of all people with diabetes, about 5–10 percent have Type I, which develops most often in children and young adults. That's why it was once called "juvenile-onset" diabetes. However, this type of diabetes can occur in people of any age.

THE PROBLEM. Type I diabetes occurs when the pancreas produces very little, if any, insulin. In short, the beta cells do not function. People with this type of diabetes are *insulin-dependent*. They must have daily doses of insulin from an outside source to function and survive. Insulin must be provided by injection with a syringe ("a shot"). It cannot be taken by mouth because the stomach acids make insulin ineffective.

THE SYMPTOMS. By understanding what happens when the body lacks insulin, you can understand the various symptoms of diabetes—the outward signs that something is wrong.

- *Lack of energy*. This symptom occurs because your body has no insulin to enable your cells to change blood sugar into energy. Without energy, you feel tired.
- *Constant hunger*. When you are unable to get energy from the sugar in your blood, your body sends out hunger signals for more food. Of course, a lack of sugar isn't the real problem. The problem is that your body can't use the sugar already there.
- *Weight loss*. This symptom often occurs because the body, unable to use sugar in the blood as a source of energy, turns to its reserve fat supplies for energy. As fat is used up, you lose weight.
- *Frequent urination* and *excessive thirst*. These symptoms are caused by a condition called *hyperglycemia*, or high blood sugar. In all people, whether they have diabetes or not, the blood circulates through the kidneys. These organs remove waste materials from the blood which are then expelled in urine. The kidneys also act like a "dam" to retain and recycle important nutrients such as sugar, sending them back into the blood. In diabetes, blood sugar rises to excessively high levels, which overwhelms the kidneys. They can't send all the sugar back into circulation, and it spills over the "dam" into the urine. Something else goes with it—water, which results in large volumes of urine. And as you lose fluids, you get extra thirsty, your body's signal to take in more fluids.
- *Blurred vision*. If you have high blood pressure, sugar can build up in the fluids of your eyes. The excess sugar draws water with it, causing the eye's outer lens to swell, which distorts your vision. However, once you begin your diabetes treatment and your blood sugar gets back to more normal levels, your vision will clear.
- *Other symptoms*. Perhaps you had other symptoms of diabetes before your problem was identified. You may have experienced *nausea, vomiting, abdominal pain, weakness*, or *rapid shallow breathing*. It's even possible you experienced a *diabetic coma* prior

to getting medical assistance. All of these symptoms can occur when your body uses stored fat instead of glucose as an alternative source of energy.

Whenever a person goes for long periods without food, it's natural for the body to use stored fat for energy. As the body uses the fat, acid substances called *ketones* are formed and accumulate in the blood. Under normal circumstances, the level of ketones is low and harmless.

In diabetes, when there is not enough insulin to allow glucose to be used for energy, the body must rely exclusively on fat for its energy needs. As a result, high levels of both glucose and ketones accumulate in the blood and spill into the urine. This process is called *ketosis* and can lead to a serious problem called *diabetic ketoacidosis*, in which the acid in the blood is excessively high. Ketoacidosis can cause all of the symptoms described above and may even lead to diabetic coma, a life-threatening condition.

THE CAUSE. Type I diabetes results from the destruction of the beta cells of the pancreas. Why does this occur? Research during the past decade has brought us closer to an answer. As yet, scientists don't know for sure, but they believe that most cases of Type I diabetes are caused when something has gone wrong in the body's *immune system*. The main job of your immune system is to fight diseases by producing *antibodies*, substances that eliminate foreign invaders, such as bacteria and viruses. In certain cases, however, the immune system goes haywire and destroys the body's own cells. Researchers believe that this is what happens in most cases of Type I diabetes. By mistake, the body destroys the beta cells of the pancreas, the very cells it needs to produce insulin.

Again, scientists don't know why this happens. But heredity probably plays a role. In other words, there is a tendency for the problem to occur more frequently in certain families. Studies show that if one parent has Type I diabetes, a child has a 5 to 10 percent chance of developing the same condition. The risk rises to 20 percent when both parents have Type I diabetes.

New tests now make it possible to detect faulty immune antibodies in the blood—years before a person shows any of the common symptoms of diabetes. In adults, the destructive antibodies may be in the blood five or more years before symptoms appear. This suggests that the destruction of beta cells doesn't occur abruptly. Instead, it is a gradual process, taking place during what is called the "prediabetic stage."

Nationwide research studies are now being undertaken to look for ways to halt the destruction of the beta cells during this stage. For this reason, people with an immediate relative with Type I diabetes are being encouraged to be tested for the presence of faulty antibodies that may lead to diabetes. If they are detected, perhaps these people can be given a treatment that would prevent further destruction of the beta cells. Insulin, itself, is one possible treatment being studied to prevent diabetes. You can contact Joslin Diabetes Center for the latest information on these prevention studies, and for information on how to be screened.

Type II: Non-Insulin-Dependent Diabetes

Type II diabetes is the most common kind of diabetes, accounting for about 90 percent of all cases. Until recently, Type II diabetes was referred to as "maturity-onset" diabetes because it occurs most often in mature adults, age 40 or older.

THE PROBLEM. If you have Type II diabetes, your beta cells can still produce insulin. But unfortunately, there isn't enough to meet the present needs of your body. Compounding the problem, your body's cells can't respond properly to the available insulin to let glucose inside. People with Type II diabetes usually do not depend on insulin injections to survive. That's why it is now often called *non-insulin-dependent* diabetes. However, it's important to note that some people with this type of diabetes may still need daily injections of insulin to maintain good health.

THE SYMPTOMS. A number of symptoms are associated with Type II diabetes, which, in many ways, are similar to those found with Type I diabetes.

- *Lack of energy*. When sugar can't enter your body's cells, they can't use it for energy, and this can lead to *fatigue*. In short, you're plumb out of energy.
- *Increased hunger*. Unable to use the available sugar for energy, the body signals for more food—what you perceive as hunger pangs.
- *Weight loss*. Unable to use the sugar in the bloodstream, the body gets its energy from stored fat. As these fat stores are used up, you lose weight.
- *Hyperglycemia*. If the body is unable to use the glucose in the bloodstream, it starts to "back up." When it accumulates to a

certain point, it creates the condition called *hyperglycemia*, or high blood sugar.

- *Blurred vision*. High blood sugar can lead to a buildup of sugar in the eye fluids. The excess sugar draws in water, causing the eye's outer lens to change shape, which distorts your vision.

- *Frequent urination and excessive thirst*. The circulating blood travels through the kidneys, where normally the unused sugar is recycled for later use or for storage. However, when the levels of blood sugar are unduly high, the kidneys are unable to recycle it all and the excess sugar spills into the urine, drawing additional water with it and resulting in large volumes of urine. This accounts for frequent urination, and depleted of its normal amount of fluids, your body sends out thirst signals, telling you to drink more fluids.

- *Irritation and damage to the nerves*. Also caused by high blood sugar, an early sign of this problem can be leg pains during the night. If this condition is allowed to continue, a serious complication called *neuropathy* may develop.

- *Suppression of the immune system*. Symptoms such as *infections* and *slow healing* often signal the onset of Type II diabetes. When blood sugar is high, the immune system becomes less effective, slowing the healing process, while cold and flu viruses, which your body can usually overcome in a relatively short time, may linger on indefinitely. In women with diabetes, suppression of the immune system can lead to vaginal infections by fungi or bacteria which may cause severe vaginal itching and can be very uncomfortable.

- *Other symptoms*. Problems with *sexual functions* are reported by men and women in both Type I and Type II diabetes. Men with diabetes are susceptible to *impotence*, the inability to achieve or maintain an erection, because high blood glucose can damage the nerves controlling the flow of blood into the penis or damage the blood vessels themselves. Women may experience sexual problems as well. Although little is known about this complication, high levels of blood glucose can cause changes or decreases in vaginal lubrication which may make intercourse painful.

- Some people discover that *mood changes* develop along with some of the other symptoms of both Type I and Type II diabetes. For example, you may feel less enthusiasm for your day-to-day activities. In reality, such mood changes are probably not caused directly by diabetes. It's more likely that the gradual loss of energy, along with the other symptoms of diabetes, may cause some people to feel unwell, which, in turn, affects their outlook on life.

THE CAUSE. Researchers do not know what causes Type II diabetes. They have determined, however, that there is no single cause. Instead, the condition seems to be brought on by a number of factors which interact in complex ways and vary from person to person:

Insulin Resistance. Insulin resistance occurs when the body "resists" taking sugar into its cells. This may happen because: (1) the insulin can't link with the receptors on the surfaces of cells because there aren't enough receptors; or (2) something goes wrong in the chemical reaction at the time of linking. In either situation, the body can't use the sugar in the blood and high blood sugar develops, bringing on the symptoms of diabetes.

Defect in the Beta Cells. In a normal pancreas, the beta cells release the right amount of insulin at the proper rate. After a meal, the surge is very rapid, and once the sugar has been used for the body's immediate energy, the rest is stored as glycogen or fat. The rate at which insulin is released then decreases, keeping blood sugar levels in the normal range of 60–140 mg/dl.

The beta cells of people with Type II diabetes are often able to secrete large amounts of insulin into the bloodstream, but for some reason these cells can't respond immediately to the rising levels of glucose. This results in a delay in the release of insulin, and by the time the beta cells get around to the job, high levels of sugar may already have built up in the blood.

Reduced Number of Beta Cells. One way to remedy the "delayed-action" situation is for the beta cells to produce more insulin. In theory, the additional insulin would then take care of the excess sugar that built up during the delay. Unfortunately, people with Type II diabetes often have fewer beta cells than normal. Even though these beta cells can make insulin, they can't make enough to handle the excess blood sugar caused by the delay.

Other Factors. Researchers don't know what causes insulin resistance or why beta cells become defective or reduced in number. However, one contributing factor is heredity—the tendency to pass on traits from one generation to the next. Studies show that if one parent has Type II diabetes, the offspring will have a 25 to 30 percent chance of developing the condition. If both parents have this type of diabetes, the risk may be as high as 50–75 percent. Additional evidence shows that if one twin develops Type II diabetes, there's a 75 percent or greater chance the other will, too. Thus, heredity is an important factor in a person's chance of having insulin resistance, defective beta cells, or a reduced number of beta cells. And sometimes, the combination of these conditions also leads to *relative insulin deficiency*. In such cases, the body produces an amount of insulin that would be enough under normal conditions. However, it's not enough to overcome insulin resistance.

Excess body weight also plays a part in insulin resistance. If you already have a genetic potential for insulin resistance, then excess weight can kick it into gear. More than 80 percent of all people diagnosed with Type II diabetes were overweight before the disease developed. By losing weight, many of these people can increase the number and efficiency of the insulin receptors in their body's cells. They still have diabetes, but by making their cells less resistant to insulin, they can gain better control of their blood sugar.

Age also is a factor in Type II diabetes. Research shows that after age 50, a larger percentage of people begin to have trouble keeping their blood sugar in normal range. After age 65, as much as 20 percent of the population has diabetes (compared with 5 percent overall). Scientists believe that as people mature, their cells are more likely to develop resistance to insulin. The aging process also causes changes in body composition. We tend to have less muscle and more fat tissue later in life, which can affect the way the body uses blood sugar.

Thus, for a variety of reasons, high blood sugar develops when your body can't produce or properly use insulin. But high blood sugar can make the problem even worse. How? Excess sugar in your blood may further damage your beta cells, making them less able to produce insulin, possibly by reducing the number of receptors on the surfaces of cells. It is a vicious cycle—the higher your blood sugar goes, the more difficult it is for the body to bring it back to normal. That's why, once diabetes has been diagnosed, it is vitally important to get it under control and keep it under control!

Other Types of Diabetes

While most people with diabetes have either Type I or Type II, there are also a few less common forms of the disease.

GESTATIONAL DIABETES. Gestation refers to the time period in which a woman is pregnant. *Gestational diabetes* is a condition in women who don't have the common form of diabetes, but for some reason can't metabolize sugar normally during their pregnancy. These women may develop a true case of diabetes after the baby is born, either right after the birth or some years later. It's important to manage gestational diabetes to avoid complications for the mother and the baby.

IMPAIRED GLUCOSE TOLERANCE. A similar condition is called *impaired glucose tolerance*. With this problem, the body's response to sugar in the blood is not normal, but it has not yet reached the level at which actual diabetes can be diagnosed. Impaired glucose tolerance can be diagnosed by giving a patient a glucose tolerance test (described below). People with this problem will show an abnormal response to the test because their bodies (1) don't produce enough insulin, (2) don't produce it fast enough, or (3) can't use the insulin properly to reduce blood sugars in a normal way. People with impaired glucose tolerance usually don't have the classic symptoms of diabetes. Even so, some may eventually develop diabetes. But for others, blood sugar levels may return to normal without treatment. However, people with this condition should take special care to maintain normal body weight and to watch for the symptoms of diabetes.

Diagnosing Diabetes

Diabetes is diagnosed in a number of ways. Often you may have some or all of the classic symptoms of diabetes. You may also have high blood sugar, which can be detected with a simple blood test. To confirm the diagnosis of diabetes, your doctor may order more than one blood test, perhaps taking a reading at different times of day.

Remember, you have glucose in your blood at all times. The question is: How much? The normal level ranges from 60–140 mg/dl if you have just eaten. A test result of more than 200 mg/dl taken one to two hours after a meal, or a fasting blood sugar level of over 140 mg/dl, is usually enough to raise strong suspicion of diabetes. However, if glucose levels are "borderline," a glucose tolerance test may be used to diagnose diabetes. In this test, you eat a large amount of carbohydrates for three days before the test. On the day of the test, having fasted since dinner the night before, your blood glucose level is measured. You then drink a glucose solution and the blood is retested at regular intervals to see how the body handles the glucose.

Urine testing is generally not used to diagnose diabetes. That's because the level of blood glucose may not be high enough to spill over into the urine—even though the level in the blood is high enough to qualify as diabetes. A test called hemoglobin A_1 (see Chapter 10) may read "high" in someone with diabetes. However, there may be reasons other than diabetes for a false reading on the hemoglobin A_1 test, for example, if a person has anemia. Therefore, experts do not recommend using this test by itself to diagnose diabetes. The person should always be tested for blood sugar levels.

After the Diagnosis

While a diagnosis of diabetes is never good news, it is not a cause for panic. But it is a cause for concern and immediate action. Once you've gained a better understanding of the causes of diabetes and how it affects your body, you must then learn what you can do to keep your body functioning as normally as possible.

CHAPTER 2

The Tools for Treatment

IF YOU HAVE BEEN diagnosed with diabetes, you may wonder: "Why do I need to know about diabetes? After all, isn't my doctor the one responsible for my treatment?" On the surface, that reaction may seem to make sense. The care provided by your health-care team is a very important part of treating diabetes. But the situation isn't that simple. To properly control your diabetes, you are the one who must be primarily responsible for the most appropriate treatment program. And once you understand the importance of a treatment program and your role in carrying it out, you're on a journey to the best health possible.

In taking that trip, you must avoid the mental detours that can rob you of your commitment. One of the biggest mistakes is thinking, "If I can't see or feel a problem, it isn't there." In diabetes, this is a dangerous notion. Many problems and complications of poorly controlled diabetes are often hidden, and for many years it may appear that everything is going fine. Only when the diabetes becomes a grave problem do you wake up to the stark reality that things have actually been amiss for a long time, and that if you had made a more positive commitment to your treatment program earlier, these problems might have been avoided.

Understanding the Basic Treatment Program

It's important to treat diabetes for two reasons. First, you want to gain relief from the immediate symptoms caused by high blood sugar. Second, your treatment can promote a state of physical well-being and vigor, and as the DCCT results mentioned earlier suggest, you can help prevent or minimize the long-term complications that can result if your blood sugar remains high for months and years.

Whatever treatment program is designed for your diabetes, the overall goal is the same—to keep your blood sugar "in control." In order to accomplish that, your treatment program will involve three basic approaches:

- *Meal planning.* This consists of the proper balance of foods and nutrients that you need to maintain good health and manage your blood sugar levels. It will also help you manage the level of fats or "lipids" in your blood, which are frequently too high in people with diabetes. Your meal plan will also take into consideration the timing of your meals in conjunction with your daily diabetes medications, goals you may have for weight loss, and the types of foods you like or dislike.
- *Regular exercise.* Exercise helps everyone, whether you have diabetes or not. Not only does it make you feel better, but it also preserves and increases muscle tone and strength, gives your heart a workout, increases lung efficiency, and helps you maintain a desired weight. If you have diabetes, you will gain an extra benefit from exercise. It enables you to use insulin better, thereby lowering the amount of sugar in your blood, generally enabling you to use smaller doses of insulin or oral medication.
- *Medications.* People with Type I diabetes need insulin injections to stay alive. People with Type II diabetes can often manage their condition with meal planning and exercise, and, sometimes, by taking pills that stimulate the body to produce additional insulin and use insulin better. But many people with Type II diabetes— those who cannot produce enough insulin—must also rely on insulin injections to bring their blood sugar into a healthy range.

Another important part of your treatment program is *monitoring,* which involves testing your blood or urine for substances that tell you how well you are managing your diabetes. All people with diabetes— both Type I and Type II—should carefully monitor the effectiveness and progress of their treatment.

To one degree or another, Type I or Type II diabetes will affect nearly all aspects of your life. That's why your treatment program should be "customized" to meet your particular needs and lifestyle. Your treatment should include *professional support* to deal with the impact of diabetes on your emotional and social well-being. You and your family should try to participate in support groups. Talk with mental health professionals about your concerns. Attend educational programs offered at your local hospital or diabetes center. By gaining the appropriate knowledge, skills, and attitudes, you will be able to manage your diabetes with competence and confidence.

Your Place in the Treatment Program

Unlike other serious illnesses, diabetes is a condition in which you must take an active part in the treatment. In fact, you will provide much of your own primary care. This doesn't mean you will be left alone to provide your own treatment. It does mean, however, that you will play an important role in the design of your treatment program. And once that treatment program has been determined, you will be the one responsible for actually carrying it out. You will have the job of maintaining and monitoring the program. And whenever you have questions or problems, you will alert your health-care team so that adjustments can be made in your meal plan, exercise program, or medication.

By taking an active role in your treatment program, you can reduce the risks of developing complications. This doesn't mean that by being totally faithful to your treatment plan you won't develop any complications. Research suggests that some people may develop complications despite their best efforts, for genetic or other inexplicable reasons. But you still will have a lot to say about preventing or slowing the long-term problems that can arise when diabetes is improperly treated. If you are faithful to a well-designed program, you are less likely to face these complications.

By actively participating in your treatment, you will also be able to achieve a far greater level of freedom and control in your everyday life. You will not have to depend on other people to carry out your daily tasks. Also, you will find it easier to cope with your concerns. Think of your treatment program as a ship. With the best equipment on board— and with the help of an experienced crew—there will be smooth sailing ahead.

The Role of the Health-Care Team

Once a diagnosis of diabetes is made, it is very important to look for a physician who is knowledgeable about the disease and its complications. As with other complex medical problems, even the best general practitioner or primary-care physician may not be aware of all of the concerns that need to be addressed in diabetes. In many medical centers, diabetes care is provided by a specially trained treatment team, which generally consists of the following professionals:

- *Diabetologist*—a physician who is an expert in treating diabetes, particularly diabetes that is treated with insulin. The physician may also be a board-certified endocrinologist (hormone specialist).

- *Nurse educator*—a nurse who is trained in the management of diabetes and is skilled in teaching procedures of diabetes care. Frequently this person is a certified diabetes educator (C.D.E.).

- *Registered dietitian*—a professional who is trained in the nutritional needs and planning of meals for people with diabetes. Many dietitians who work with diabetes patients are also C.D.E.s.

- *Exercise physiologist*—a person trained to help people with diabetes devise an effective exercise program.

- *Mental health specialist*—someone who can help you and your family deal with the emotional and social impact of a chronic condition such as diabetes.

- *Other professionals*—include ophthalmologists (eye doctors) and podiatrists (foot doctors).

In addition to providing expert medical care, such a team can give you insights on a host of issues that relate to the care and management of your diabetes. They can assist you with your particular concerns and situations, including the effect of diabetes on your work or family life. The team is also prepared to show you how a wide range of available resources—advances in treatment, the care of other professionals, a proper outlook on your part, and the assistance of family and friends— can help you deal more successfully with your diabetes. Among the additional resources you may need are specialists who deal with specific complications of diabetes, for example, an *ophthalmologist* (eye doctor) or *nephrologist* (kidney specialist). In fact, if you have diabetes, you should have your eyes examined yearly. Your health-care team may refer you to these specialists, when needed, to either prevent or treat such complications.

Most people turn to their diabetes treatment team for help managing their diabetes while continuing to see their primary-care physician for their other medical needs. The diabetes team works with the patient, and the patient's primary-care physician, to develop and monitor the individualized treatment plan.

It's comforting to know that a team of experts is ready to assist you. But remember, you are the most important member of the crew. You are the person who ultimately will be responsible for steering the ship to safe harbor.

Part Two

TREATING DIABETES WITH NUTRITION AND EXERCISE

CHAPTER 3

Eating with Diabetes

IF YOU HAVE DIABETES, your body is having trouble getting energy from the food you eat. That's why it is important for you to know something about the nutritional value of food. You then can use that knowledge to devise a meal plan that will both provide the proper nutrition and help keep your blood sugar in control. You will also enjoy the additional benefit of being able to eat the kinds of food you like without feeling deprived.

We all need to maintain a healthy diet, and the U.S. Department of Health and Human Services has issued the following dietary guidelines for everyone to follow:

- Eat a variety of foods.
- Maintain desirable weight.
- Avoid too much overall fat in your diet, particularly saturated fat and cholesterol.
- Eat foods with adequate starch and fiber.
- Avoid eating too much sugar.
- Avoid too much sodium (found in table salt). Beware of processed and "fast foods" with high salt content.
- If you drink alcoholic beverages, do so in moderation.

If you have diabetes, you need to follow one more important guideline:

- *You should be extra careful about the foods you eat to keep your blood sugar in a normal range.*

Why Does Meal Planning Matter?

When you go on a vacation, you use a map to help guide you to your destination. You also plan special activities to make your trip a success. In like manner, if you have diabetes, you should follow a meal plan. It is your nutritional "road map" that will help you keep your blood sugar in normal range.

To devise and follow a meal plan, you simply select and eat foods that will help you to best manage your diabetes. These foods are not unfamiliar or special. They include many items you ate before you discovered you had diabetes. But there are special precautions you should take in planning your meals:

- Notice the kind of food you eat: for example, focus on foods that are low in saturated fat.
- Watch how much you eat.
- If you take insulin, coordinate your food intake with the action of the insulin.
- Limit foods high in sugar, as these can quickly use up the amount of carbohydrate you are able to eat as part of your meal plan.

Timing Is Everything

The basic strategy behind your meal plan is to coordinate your food intake with the action of the insulin in your body. It won't do your cells much good to have blood sugar "knocking on the door" if there is no insulin "key" to let it in. That's why a meal planning approach may be recommended for both Type I and Type II diabetes patients. But no two cases are exactly alike, so your meal plan must be tailored to your particular condition.

For example, if you have Type I diabetes, you must use insulin injections to replace the insulin no longer produced by the pancreas. This insulin will act at specific times after it is injected, and these action times will vary, depending on the type of insulin you use (short-acting, intermediate-acting, and long-acting). Your meal plan must coordinate with these action times. If you have Type II diabetes and take insulin to supplement the small amount of insulin still produced by your pancreas, or if you take pills to boost insulin production or improve your body's ability to use insulin, many of these same concerns apply. Either way, your food intake still must be timed to coincide with your own insulin production and not to overwhelm it.

The timing of food intake with the action of insulin is important for everyone with diabetes. The question is not whether you have Type I or Type II diabetes. The main question is: *When is the insulin in your body acting?* This will determine, in part, *when* and *how much* you will be able to eat.

Insulin acts upon the blood sugar circulating in your bloodstream. That sugar comes from the food you eat. It also comes from other sources, such as the sugar stored in your body. To get the most out of your meal plan, you must carefully coordinate the amount and time you eat with the peak time that your insulin is acting. The idea is to match as closely as possible each side of this equation:

Sugar in bloodstream = Sugar that the insulin in your blood-stream can handle

Benefits and Rewards

In following a meal plan, you stand to gain the short- and long-term benefits that come with maintaining your blood sugar at the proper level. You will feel better and have more energy. Also, for certain people with Type II diabetes, a meal plan can help reduce *insulin resistance*. This condition develops when the body's cells "resist" the action of available insulin. Insulin resistance is linked to heredity and excess weight, so if you shed extra pounds, your cells will be better able to use insulin. A meal plan can help you lose weight, which helps reduce insulin resistance. But just eating the right amount and variety of foods at the right time will also help your body combat insulin resistance, before you even lose a single pound.

Meal planning can help combat two other factors associated with Type II diabetes—*defective beta cells* and a *reduced number of beta cells* in the pancreas. When you follow a meal plan, your beta cells will be able to respond more quickly to your body's needs for your insulin, such as immediately after a meal. You may still need to use injected insulin to boost your body's natural insulin production, but the dose may be much smaller.

Fighting Complications

People who have had diabetes for many years are susceptible to serious complications, some that can even be life-threatening. In years past, your chances of developing such complications were high. Following a meal plan can help avert that risk for people with both Type I and Type II diabetes. And you will have the confidence of knowing that you're doing everything you can to prevent the long-term complications that may arise with poorly controlled diabetes. As the Diabetes Control and Complications Trial demonstrated, there is evidence that you can reduce the risks of complications by maintaining your blood sugar at normal or near-normal levels. A meal plan is an important part of this effort. Or if you have already developed some complications from your diabetes, following a meal plan can work to slow their progression.

In addition to helping you keep your blood sugar in control, a meal plan is based on sound principles of nutrition. By following these principles, you will reduce the health risks that come with diets high in saturated fat, salt, and cholesterol. Foods high in these substances increase the risk of heart and blood vessel disease, and people with diabetes are more likely to develop these problems than people who do not have the disease. A meal plan will help you ward off these problems and stay healthier.

CREATING A MEAL PLAN

In creating a meal plan, don't think of it as a "diet." That term usually implies a drastic and temporary eating strategy often used to lose weight. Instead, your goal is to develop a healthy and lifelong "eating style" that will help you combat diabetes as well as contribute to your optimum health.

In designing a meal plan, you should consult with a registered dietitian who is an expert in nutrition. You and your dietitian will consider a number of factors in creating a meal plan. More than just the food you eat, the factors include:

- *Lifestyle.* What is your work schedule? Do you exercise?
- *Medication.* Are you taking insulin? Pills? If so, how much and when does the action of your medication peak?
- *Weight goals.* Do you need to gain weight? Lose weight? Maintain your current weight?
- *Medical condition.* Do you have any other medical problems that may affect what you should or should not eat?
- *Food preferences.* What kinds of food do you like? Are you a vegetarian?

In designing a customized meal plan to meet your individual needs, your dietitian may fill out a special form similar to Figure 3-1 for an exchange meal plan. Let's look at this in detail.

Names and Phone Number

Near the top of the Meal Plan form is a place for your name as well as the name and telephone number of your dietitian. If you have questions about the foods you eat, do not hesitate to contact your dietitian.

Calories

Also in the top section (right column) is a space labeled "Calories." A calorie is a way of measuring the amount of energy supplied by food. Your dietitian will indicate the approximate number of calories your body needs each day to balance the calories you burn. The amount is determined by your height, weight, age, sex, and level of activity. If you need to lose weight, the number of calories will be reduced so that you burn more calories than you eat.

Carbohydrate, Protein, and Fat

Alongside the space for calories are three spaces labeled CHO, PRO, and FAT—the abbreviations for carbohydrate, protein, and fat. These are the nutrients your body uses to produce energy, build and repair body tissue, and regulate body functions. Your dietitian will write the number of grams of these nutrients you should include in your daily meal plan. This is determined by the number of calories you need. Carbohydrate and protein provide 4 calories per gram; fat provides 9 calories per gram.

Food Groups

The rest of this Meal Plan form is divided into two vertical columns titled "Meal" and "Sample Menu." Look first at the left-hand column titled "Meal." It lists three daily meals—breakfast, lunch, and dinner.

Under the heading for each meal are the six food groups into which all foods are divided—Milk, Vegetable, Fruit, Bread/Starch, Meat, and Fat. (Note only five groups are listed for breakfast; it has no vegetable portion.) This form is an example of an exchange meal plan.

FIGURE 3-1. MEAL PLAN FORM

MEAL PLAN

Dietitian _____ Name _____

Phone _____ Date _____

CHO _____ FAT _____

PRO _____ Calories _____

MEAL	SAMPLE MENU
BREAKFAST Time _____ *Number of Choices*	
_____ Milk	_____
_____ Fruit	_____
_____ Bread/Starch	_____
_____ Meat	_____
_____ Fat	_____
MORNING SNACK Time _____	
LUNCH Time _____ *Number of Choices*	
_____ Milk	_____
_____ Vegetable	_____
_____ Fruit	_____
_____ Bread/Starch	_____
_____ Meat	_____
_____ Fat	_____
AFTERNOON SNACK Time _____	
DINNER Time _____ *Number of Choices*	
_____ Milk	_____
_____ Vegetable	_____
_____ Fruit	_____
_____ Bread/Starch	_____
_____ Meat	_____
_____ Fat	_____
EVENING SNACK Time _____	

Food Choices in an Exchange Meal Plan

In the spaces to the left of the food groups, your dietitian will write the "Number of Choices" of foods you may have from each food group for breakfast, lunch, and dinner. What is a choice? It is a measured amount of food that contains an average number of grams of carbohydrate, protein, or fat (often a combination of all three nutrients). Each choice provides an average number of calories. Refer to the Appendix, Food Choice Lists. At the left of each item on the lists and a measured portion of that item, you will find the average number of grams of carbohydrate, protein, and fat it provides, along with the number of calories in that portion.

The type and number of choices you have will depend, in part, on how many calories you require. An active person who needs 2,500 calories will have more choices than someone in a weight-loss program who needs only 1,200–1,500 calories.

Once your dietitian has determined the number of choices you may have from each food group, he or she will write out a sample menu, like the one found in the right-hand column of the Meal Plan form.

HOW TO USE AN EXCHANGE MEAL PLAN

There is a lot of flexibility built into an exchange meal plan. The items listed in the Food Choice Lists are an indication of the variety of foods you may choose for an actual meal. And you can "exchange" one food for another according to your preference and tastes. For example, if your meal plan calls for one vegetable choice, you may exchange ½ cup of broccoli for 1 cup of green beans. Notice that a portion value is assigned to each item on the Food Choice Lists. This is no accident. These values have been calculated so that each item will provide you with equal amounts of calories and nutrients and will affect your blood sugar in a similar way. For that reason, you can interchange items within a food choice.

Overall, the beauty of a meal plan is that it offers both *flexibility* and *sameness*. You have a wide range of food items for every choice. Yet by sticking to the number of choices on your meal plan, you actually will be eating about the same amount of carbohydrate, protein, and fat at each meal every day. That is very important in managing your diabetes. People who do not have diabetes can vary their food intake because their pancreas automatically adjusts the level of insulin. By contrast, many people with diabetes usually take a prescribed amount of insulin at certain times of the day. Your health-care team bases the dose and timing on the amount of food in your meal plan and your average level of physical activity.

What happens if you don't stick to your meal plan? If you eat more than your meal plan allows, there will be too much sugar in your bloodstream for the insulin to handle. The result: your blood sugar will be higher than normal. If you don't eat enough, you will have too much insulin. The result: your blood sugar will be lower than normal. To keep your blood sugar within normal range, you should keep your food intake nearly the same from one day to the next, unless you are using an intensive diabetes therapy program, in which you are adjusting your medication on a daily basis in response to your blood sugar testing results. See Chapter 9 for more information on this program.

Time of Day

For each meal and snack, your dietitian will indicate the time of day to eat. It's very important that you eat each meal at about the same time every day. Sticking to such a schedule may be quite different from your previous eating habits. Before you had diabetes, your pancreas was on "automatic." It could maintain a normal range of blood sugar by slowly secreting insulin. And when you needed extra insulin, for example, at meals, the pancreas would respond with a burst of insulin. The extra insulin helped your body's cells to use the additional blood sugar for energy or to store it for future use.

Now that you have diabetes, you no longer have a precise, automatic system to handle the sugar in your blood. If you are taking insulin, the dose prescribed by your doctor usually consists of a combination of various types. Each type has these features:

- *Onset*—the period of time insulin takes to begin working
- *Peak activity*—when insulin is most effective
- *Duration*—the length of time of insulin's activity, including its tapering-off time

Your insulin should be timed to correspond with your usual intake of food. Or your intake of food must be timed to correspond with the actions of your insulin. If you choose the latter, you must eat meals at the same times each day to match your insulin schedule. (This topic is discussed at length in Chapter 8.) If you are using intensive diabetes therapy, and therefore are closely monitoring your blood sugar throughout the day, you may have more flexibility in the timing of your meals and your medication. (This will be discussed in Chapter 9.)

Snacks

Let's look again at the Meal Plan form. You will notice spaces for snacks between meals and also at bedtime. These snacks are often essential for you to maintain blood sugar levels as close to normal as possible. Your need for a snack is related to the way insulin is released into your bloodstream. Once injected, insulin is released from the injection site into your blood, and it continues to act even after the sugar from a meal has been used. So if you have not eaten recently, there may not be enough sugar for the insulin to act upon. In such a case, the continuing action of insulin may reduce the blood sugar to levels below normal.

This condition is called low blood sugar or *hypoglycemia*. To prevent low blood sugar, you may have to snack between meals or at bedtime.

CARBOHYDRATE COUNTING

There are other types of meal planning techniques that are increasingly being used by people with diabetes and their health-care team. One of these is called *carbohydrate counting*, which can be used by people on intensive therapy or those employing more traditional forms of diabetes management.

Carbohydrate counting has become more popular since the American Diabetes Association liberalized its eating guidelines for people with diabetes in 1994. At that time, a committee of the ADA observed that there was little scientific evidence to support efforts to restrict people with diabetes from eating sugar-containing foods. They noted that 10 grams of carbohydrate will have basically the same effect on a person's blood sugar, whether its source is table sugar or potatoes. What is important is how much total carbohydrate you eat—regardless of the source.

The concepts behind carbohydrate counting reflect this change in thinking. If you choose this form of meal planning, your dietitian will determine the total number of grams of carbohydrate you should eat at a given meal or snack, based on your medication and exercise patterns, your weight loss goals if you have any, etc. It will then be your choice as to how you fulfill those carbohydrate needs. You'll probably have to buy a carbohydrate-counting book, which can be found in many bookstores and even at some supermarket checkouts.

Here's how carbohydrate counting works. Your dietitian may calculate that you usually eat 75 grams of carbohydrate at dinner, for example. One night you may choose to eat those 75 grams in the form of 1 cup of cooked rice (45 grams of carbohydrate), 1 cup of milk (12 grams of carbohydrate) and ½ cup of applesauce (15 grams of carbohydrate). Another night you might decide to skip the applesauce, cut back to ⅔ of a cup of rice (30 grams of carbohydrate), and drink that milk (12 grams) with a small piece of angel food cake, which has 30 grams of carbohydrate.

Of course, you won't want to substitute sweets for more healthy foods at every meal—no one should, whether you have diabetes or not. Also, you need to note how much fat may be in a sweet that you are substituting in a given meal—if weight loss is a goal, or you have high blood fat levels, you don't want to add lots of fat to your diet. But, thanks to the new guidelines, you needn't feel deprived. All things in moderation.

These new guidelines and the use of carbohydrate counting can be particularly helpful for children and teens with diabetes—it will help them join in with friends when social occasions include eating. But parents should be wary of letting their children use up their carbohydrate allotments with soft drinks and candy which lack any nutritional value.

FAT-GRAM COUNTING

Another way you and your dietitian may choose to attack the issue of how to eat well while managing your diabetes may be by using the concepts behind fat-gram counting. As you can perhaps imagine, in this scenario you are counting the grams of fat you are eating, rather than, or in addition to, the grams of carbohydrate. This is particularly important if you are trying to lose weight. More on fat-gram counting appears in Chapter 6.

Questions About Eating with Diabetes

Here are some questions that people with diabetes commonly ask about exchange meal plans and other eating programs that they use as part of their diabetes management program.

Q. *If I use an exchange meal plan, can I omit some of the choices for a particular meal? For example, if I prefer a light breakfast, can I use some of the breakfast choices for lunch or dinner?*

A. No, this is not a good idea unless you are doing your own insulin adjustments as part of an intensified program (see Chapter 9). All food choices are scheduled throughout the day to help maintain normal levels of blood sugar. For example, it was once thought that you could save fat choices and move them from one meal to the next. However, dietary fats can help slow the rise of blood sugar after a meal, so it's better not to switch them.

Q. *For a particular meal, can I use all my choices in a single food group on one item of food? For example, if my breakfast lists two bread/starch choices, can they both be used for English muffins, rather than for two different items?*

A. Yes. However, different foods contain different nutrients, so it's better to have as much variety in your food choices as possible.

Q. *Can I substitute a choice in one food group for a choice in another group if they both provide about the same amount of carbohydrate, protein, and fat? For example, can I substitute a bread/starch choice for a fruit choice?*

A. Yes. You should heed the following suggestions, however:

Substitutions Between Food Groups

- Replace one (1) fruit choice with one (1) bread/starch choice. Try to limit this substitution to no more than once a day. Otherwise, you will eliminate the vitamins A and C present in fruit.
- Replace one (1) bread/starch choice with three (3) vegetable choices. Use this substitution to provide yourself with more fiber and "bulk" when you're especially hungry.

- Replace one (1) skim or 1% low-fat milk choice with one (1) bread/starch choice and one (1) low-fat meat choice. This substitution should be made only occasionally, or you will eliminate the calcium present in milk from your meal plan.

STUDYING THE "FOOD MAP"

Again, we encourage you to think of meal planning as a nutritional road map. But to more fully understand the direction you are headed, it's important to learn a few more facts about food.

CHAPTER 4

More Food Facts

Before a carpenter can build a house, he first must learn some basic facts about building materials. He then learns how they all fit together into the framework of a building. In similar fashion, it's important for you to know the basics about food and nutrition. You can then use that knowledge to develop a healthy eating style through your meal plan—one that will help keep your blood sugar in normal range.

Nature's Building Blocks

All the foods we eat are made up of *nutrients*, the substances that provide the body what it needs to grow, stay warm, and provide a wide range of other functions. In short, what we need to live! The three major nutrients that are traditionally of concern for someone with diabetes are *carbohydrates*, *protein*, and *fat*. In addition, research suggests that other nutrients—certain vitamins and minerals—may also be important in the care of diabetes. More about that later. First, however, let's talk about carbohydrates, protein, and fat.

Carbohydrates

Commonly known as sugars and starches, carbohydrates are the body's main source of energy. There are two basic types of carbohydrates: *simple* and *complex*. Simple carbohydrates are commonly called sugars. When we think of sugar, we often think only of the fine white grains of table sugar. But there actually are dozens of types of sugar. For example, names of sugars include *lactose* (found in milk), *glucose* and *fructose* (found in fruit and vegetables), and *sucrose* (also called cane or beet sugar). This, of course, means that "sugar" under a variety of names can be found in a wide range of foods—candy, sugar-sweetened beverages and fruit drinks, milk, fruits and vegetables, sugar-coated cereals, honey, syrup, preserves, and desserts of all kinds.

Complex carbohydrates are just that—complex. They are made up of large numbers of sugar molecules (glucose) joined together in a long chain. Complex carbohydrates are found in all the starches that we eat, such as bread, pasta, rice, beans, potatoes, corn, peas, carrots, beets, and broccoli. In addition, all types of fiber are complex carbohydrates. Whole grains, fruits, and vegetables are good sources of fiber. However, fiber is the indigestible part of plants, and therefore contributes no calories. But as you will learn later, fiber is important for proper body function.

The body breaks down most carbohydrates—whether simple or complex—into a simple sugar called glucose. Both sugars and starches are broken down or digested into glucose at about the same speed, so it is important to control all the different carbohydrates you eat, not just the sugars. The glucose is released into the bloodstream and circulated to the cells of your body. The cells then use this glucose for energy or store it for future use. For many years people thought complex carbohydrates break down more slowly than simple ones. As the new American Diabetes Association recommendations state, research has never shown this to be the case. Therefore, the glucose from complex carbohydrates is absorbed into the blood at about the same rate as that from simple carbohydrates. That's why people with diabetes should watch how much both simple and complex carbohydrates they eat.

Protein

Protein is the second major nutrient needed by your body. The word *protein* is derived from a Greek word meaning "of first importance," which is indicative of protein's role as the basic building material of life. Your body uses protein primarily to build and repair body tissue. Muscles, organs, bones, skin, and many of the chemical messengers in your body are made of protein. Protein can also provide energy for your body if carbohydrates are not available.

Protein is not a simple substance. It is a chain of building blocks called *amino acids*. In the human body, there are 22 amino acids, and they combine with each other in an almost infinite number of arrangements. Plants and some bacteria can manufacture all the amino acids they need. But the human body can make only 13 of the 22 amino acids it needs for survival, so 9 of the amino acids must come from an outside source—the food you eat. You can get these amino acids by eating plant protein or by eating the meat from animals that consumed protein. Protein is found in food such as meat, poultry, fish, eggs, cheese, and milk. Grain, legumes, and nuts also contain protein, with other sources including foods such as oatmeal, lentils, and peanuts.

Fat

The third nutrient your body needs is fat. That's right, your body needs fat! Contrary to what you may have been led to believe in diet ads, fat is not all bad. It's only when we eat too much fat or the wrong kind that it becomes a problem. Fat is an oily or greasy material, and it is found in either solid or liquid form. It is prevalent in marbled meat, dairy products such as whole milk, butter, and cheese, margarine, and vegetable oils such as corn, sunflower, and olive oil.

Fat is used by the body in a number of ways. It's important for maintaining healthy skin and hair. Fat also serves as a "vehicle" to carry fat-soluble vitamins throughout your body. In addition, fats are changed by the body into fatty acids—an important source of energy for the muscles and heart. Fat is also used to store energy. Any extra calories produced from the carbohydrates, protein, or fat that your body does not use immediately are stored in the body as body fat (*adipose tissue*).

EFFECT OF FOOD ON DIABETES

The old adage "You are what you eat" applies to all people, whether they have diabetes or not. But it takes on special meaning for people with diabetes. That's because the types of food you eat and when you eat can have a dramatic effect on your blood sugar. Food can also be a factor in the prevention of long-term complications from diabetes.

Effect on Blood Sugar

Each of the various kinds of nutrients affects your blood sugar in different ways. Carbohydrates raise the level of blood sugar more rapidly than protein or fat. If you have diabetes, should you completely avoid sugar? First of all, that is nearly impossible because sucrose is the leading food additive used in the United States. But being cautious about the simple sugars you eat is good advice. That means eating sucrose only within the context of a healthful diet. Recent research shows that the effect of carbohydrates on your blood sugar depends on the *total amount* of complex and simple carbohydrates in your diet. The effect varies from person to person, however, so it's a good idea to consult with your health-care team about balancing the simple and complex carbohydrates in your diet.

Fat and Cholesterol

Let's first look at the effect of dietary fat on diabetes. Although the treatment of diabetes primarily involves managing sugar in the blood, the types and amounts of fat you eat can play a major role in the development of heart disease, stroke, or hardening of the arteries (*athero-sclerosis*), which is also an important concern. If you have diabetes, you have a much higher risk of developing these problems than people who do not have diabetes. To reduce those risks, both you and your doctor will want to pay attention to the levels of fat in your bloodstream.

Also, a high-fat diet is one of the main reasons people are overweight. That's because fat packs a double punch of calories into every gram. A gram of fat contains nearly 9 calories, compared with only 4 calories for every gram of carbohydrates or protein. Being overweight is something people with diabetes should avoid. Those extra pounds put a strain on your heart and also make your body's cells more resistant to insulin.

How much fat is too much? If you are overweight, you probably have been asked to limit your fat intake. If you have abnormally high levels of blood fats (lipids), you may also be asked to modify the types and amounts of fats you eat. Don't feel bad. You're not being singled out. These guidelines are suggested for *everyone*. Most of us eat way too much fat—we all need to cut back.

Saturated vs. Unsaturated Fat

There actually are two different types of dietary fat: *saturated fat* and *unsaturated fat* (both polyunsaturated and monounsaturated). Saturated fat comes from animal products, such as meat, eggs, and dairy products. It is generally "solid" at room temperatures, with the exception of the tropical oils (palm oil and coconut oil). Unsaturated fat comes from vegetables and usually is "liquid" at room temperatures—for example, corn, sunflower, safflower, canola, and olive oils.

Cholesterol

Fat and cholesterol are often mentioned together. Cholesterol is not a fat, but it does act in connection with fats in the body. Cholesterol is a waxlike substance that gets into your bloodstream in several ways. It can be manufactured by the liver and the intestines. Or it can enter the body through the foods you eat. Cholesterol is found in animal products such as fatty red meats, egg yolks, and whole-milk dairy products.

If your body has too much cholesterol, it is deposited on the walls of your arteries, which causes them to close down or clog completely. In short, you become a good candidate for a heart attack or stroke. To reduce your risk of cardiovascular disease, you should limit the amount of cholesterol you eat to no more than 300 milligrams per day. The amount of dietary cholesterol found in most products is listed on the product labels.

There are two types of cholesterol made by your body—good and bad. LDL (which stands for *low-density lipoprotein*) is considered "bad" because it is deposited into the arteries. On the other hand, HDL (*high-density lipoprotein*) is considered "good" because it actually sweeps cholesterol from the arteries and carries it back to the liver, where it is reprocessed or eliminated.

Let's look again at saturated and unsaturated fat. Each of these fats acts in concert with the two types of cholesterol. Saturated fat is considered unhealthy because it raises the level of bad (LDL) cholesterol in your bloodstream, making you more susceptible to clogged arteries. By contrast, unsaturated fat is thought to help prevent heart and vessel disease. How? Researchers believe unsaturated fats work to lower the amount of bad cholesterol. In fact, unsaturated fats may even help raise the level of good (HDL) cholesterol. But this does not mean you should go overboard on eating unsaturated fat.

You now understand why unsaturated fats are recommended over saturated fats. You should aim to keep the level of "good" HDL in your bloodstream over 35 mg/dl. The "bad" LDL should be under 130 mg/dl if you have no history of heart or artery disease. You can help this process by eating foods low in cholesterol and by getting most of your fat in the form of unsaturated fat. Exercise also helps increase levels of good cholesterol.

Because you have diabetes, your doctor will recommend certain tests to see if your levels of HDLs and LDLs are hitting these targets. This is because you are more likely to have problems with HDL and LDL levels than nondiabetics and are more likely to develop heart and artery disease as a result.

Triglycerides

People with diabetes also need to be concerned with levels of *triglycerides*, a type of storage fat in your body. High levels of triglycerides are linked with an increased risk of heart and blood vessel disease in people with diabetes. If you didn't have diabetes, your doctor would tell you to keep your triglycerides in your blood at no more than 200 mg/dl, measured when you are fasting. For people with a higher than normal risk of heart or vascular (blood vessel) disease (and that includes anyone with diabetes), triglyceride levels should be no higher than 150 mg/dl.

High blood sugar will increase triglyceride levels. To lower the levels of triglycerides in your bloodstream, you should reduce your intake of carbohydrates. Also, shed those extra pounds, exercise regularly, and avoid alcohol.

To develop a healthy eating program involving fat, specialists advise a three-pronged approach: reduce total fat intake, substitute unsaturated fat for saturated fat, and limit your intake of dietary cholesterol to no more than 300 milligrams per day. Your dietitian can help you decide the best way to lower fat and cholesterol in your diet. Here are some options:

Tips to Reduce Fat and Cholesterol

- Avoid high-fat, high-cholesterol foods. These include animal-based foods such as red meats, eggs, whole milk, butter, or whole-milk cheeses. Instead, drink skim milk or skim-milk products. Use tub margarine with liquid oil as the primary ingredient in place of butter or sour cream.
- Stock your refrigerator with foods that are naturally low-fat and cholesterol-free, like fresh fruits and vegetables.
- When cooking poultry, remove the skin. Or cook with the skin on, but don't eat it.
- Bake, broil, roast, boil, or steam foods, rather than frying.
- Use nonstick cooking sprays, which are low in calories. Or use a small dab of margarine in a nonstick pan. Avoid lard, bacon fat, and shortening.

- When preparing recipes, experiment by cutting the fat by one-fourth or one-third. For example, if a muffin recipe calls for 1 cup of oil, try ¾. If that works, next time try ⅔ cup.
- When a recipe calls for milk, use skim milk or 1% low-fat milk. If the result is too thin, try evaporated skim milk, which also can be used effectively in cream soups and can be whipped when partially frozen.
- Remove the fats from gravy and soup, using a fat separator (a small pitcher with a specially designed spout). Or refrigerate the food overnight and skim off the fat when hardened.
- In recipes, substitute low-fat or nonfat plain yogurt for sour cream. To help prevent separation in cooked foods, blend a small amount of flour or cornstarch (1 tablespoon) into the yogurt.
- For half or all of the ground beef required in a recipe, substitute ground white turkey or ground white chicken meat.
- Eat no more than 2 to 4 eggs per week. Each large egg has about 213 milligrams of cholesterol. In recipes, use an egg white for one whole egg, or use egg substitutes like Fleischmann's Egg Beaters.

Another way to reduce fat is to use products that contain *fat substitutes* or *fat replacers*. Most fat replacers are made from all-natural, food-based substances. They fall into three categories:

- *Carbohydrate-based*, which are excellent thickeners and stabilizers and are used in many formulated foods, such as margarine, mayonnaise, and baked desserts.
- *Protein-based*, which are good for frozen and refrigerated products, such as dairy products, cream-type products, and prepared entrees such as pizza.
- *Fat-based*, which, after being chemically altered, have fewer calories than fat or no calories at all. These are very stable when heated and, therefore, are good for use in frying.

For example, the product called Simplesse is a protein-based substitute made of sugar and proteins from egg white and milk, whipped into a creamy emulsion to add bulk. This product is used in frozen desserts, dips, and other products. But like the sugar-substitute aspartame, Simplesse cannot be used for cooking or frying because it clumps together, similar to an egg white when heated. Simplesse products offer a few less calories than regular products, but significantly less fat. However, you need to be careful in using products containing this fat substitute—they also may contain sugar, so eat only a small portion. And remember to ask your dietitian how to calculate the carbohydrate into your overall diet.

Fiber

Fiber is a carbohydrate that comes from whole grains, vegetables, fruits, nuts, and seeds. It is the part of the plant that cannot be digested or absorbed by your body. Therefore, fiber does not provide calories. But it does add "bulk" to your meals, helping you feel full.

There are two different types of fiber. *Water-insoluble* fiber does not dissolve in water. It helps the digestive tract function well, moving wastes through the intestines. It may prevent or relieve constipation. Wheat bran is this type of fiber and can be found in bran flakes, bran muffins, and whole-wheat bread.

Water-soluble fiber dissolves in water. In doing so, it becomes a "gummy gel" that slows the passage of food from the stomach to the intestines. This form of fiber is particularly good for people with diabetes because it may help lower their cholesterol level.

Here are ways you can increase the fiber content of your meals:

- Select whole-grain breads and cereals, instead of refined flour products.
- Sprinkle 1 tablespoon of unprocessed bran, bran cereal, oat bran, or wheat germ over fresh salads, unsweetened applesauce, hot cereal, and cottage cheese.
- Use oatmeal instead of bread crumbs in recipes.
- Include fruits and vegetables with skins whenever possible: for example, skins of baked potatoes and unpeeled apples.
- Eat dried beans and other legumes.
- Drink 6 to 8 glasses of water each day to help your body use fiber effectively.

Sugar

Used in large amounts, dietary sugar can cause an abnormally high rise in blood sugar. That's because carbohydrates are digested rapidly in the intestinal tract and become glucose, which allows them to enter the bloodstream quickly. If you do not have enough insulin in your bloodstream to handle this surge, your blood sugar levels could rise too high.

The following foods have a high sugar content and may cause problems with your diabetes management. If you are using carbohydrate counting as part of your eating plan, you may be able to use these techniques to incorporate some of these foods into your meals.

HIGH-SUGAR FOODS. Foods that are high in sugar are often also high in fat and calories. They may contribute little else of nutritional value and are best avoided until you have met with your dietitian to discuss their use. You will notice on the Food Choice Lists at the end of the book that the portion sizes for foods that contain sugar are much lower than their low-sugar alternatives. For example:

sugar-free yogurt—1 cup	*versus*	regular fruited yogurt—⅓ cup
lite pancake syrup—2 tbsp	*versus*	regular pancake syrup—1 tbsp

There are times that your physician or dietitian may recommend some of these high-carbohydrate foods to treat low blood sugar or on sick days (see Chapter 13).

The following foods should be avoided until you meet with a dietitian and learn if and how they can be included in your meal plan.

Alcohol*: sweet wines, liqueurs, cordials
Candy
Carbonated beverages with sugar, including "regular" soda
Cereals (sugar-coated)
Chewing gum (regular)
Dates, figs, and other dried fruits
Desserts containing sugar
    Cake
    Cookies with filling or frosting
    Ice cream, including sodas, shakes, and sundaes
    Ice milk
    Gelatin dessert, sweetened
    Pie

---

*Alcohol may interfere with the management of your diabetes. Always consult with your physician or dietitian before using it. See pages 279–282 for more information on the effect of alcohol in the care of diabetes.

    Pudding
    Sherbet
Fructose
Fruited yogurt
Honey
Jam and jelly (nondietetic)
Marmalade
Pastries
Preserves
Special "dietetic" foods
Sugar
Sugar-sweetened fruit drinks (Kool-Aid, Hi-C, etc.)
Sweetened condensed milk
Syrups (maple, molasses, etc.)

Types of Sugar and Sweeteners

If you have diabetes, you don't have to give up the "sweet life" entirely. There is a wide range of sweeteners available today that will fit into your eating program. But not all sweeteners are alike—they can have a different effect on your blood glucose and blood fat (lipid) levels. Table 4-1, Sugars, Sweeteners, and Sweets, is designed to assist you in understanding the different types that are available.

The table lists most of the sweeteners available today—their brand names, common names, and the "alias" by which they are known. Nonnutritive sweeteners have no calories and can be used by children and adults. It is recommended that you avoid saccharin if you are pregnant.

Sweeteners that contain calories (called nutritive sweeteners) will affect your blood sugar. These sweeteners are all carbohydrates and contain 4 calories per gram. Certain amounts of these sweeteners may be incorporated into your meals, but it is very important to control the portions. Your dietitian can explain to you how to do this, depending on whether you are using exchange meal planning, carbohydrate counting, or other meal planning techniques.

Nonnutritive sweeteners contain few, if any, calories and are therefore called *noncaloric* sweeteners. These will have no effect on your blood sugar, so people with diabetes can use these types of sweeteners. You will discover that different artificial sweeteners have different cooking properties and tastes, so you may want to try a variety, depending on the way you plan to use them.

TABLE 4-1. SUGARS, SWEETENERS, AND SWEETS

NONNUTRITIVE (NONCALORIC) SWEETENER	ALIAS	COMMENTS/APPLICATIONS
Aspartame	Equal Spoonfuls Sweetmate	180 times sweeter than sucrose. Loses sweetening effect when heated. Not acceptable for use in baking/cooking. Acceptable for use during pregnancy.
Saccharin	Sucaryl Sugar Twin Sweet Magic Sweet 'N Low Zero-Cal	375 times sweeter than sucrose. Can be used in baking and cooking.
Acesulfame-K	Sweet One Swiss Sweet	200 times sweeter than sucrose. Can be used in baking and cooking.

NUTRITIVE (CALORIC) SWEETENER	ALIAS	COMMENTS/APPLICATIONS
Carob	Carob flour Carob powder Carob tips	75% sucrose, glucose, and/or fructose. Tastes like chocolate.
Chocolate	Bittersweet Bitter, Milk chocolate	40%–43% sucrose.
Fructose	Fruit sugar Levulose	100% fruit sugar.
Glucose	Corn sugar Dextrose Grape sugar	Not as sweet as sucrose.
Honey	Creamed honey Honeycomb	About 35% glucose, 40% fructose plus water.
Lactose	Milk sugar	50% glucose. Not as sweet as sucrose.
Maltose		100% glucose. Not as sweet as sucrose.

TABLE 4-1. (continued)

NUTRITIVE (CALORIC) SWEETENER	ALIAS	COMMENTS/APPLICATIONS
Molasses	Black strap Golden syrup Refiner's sugar	50%–75% sucrose and invert sugar.
Sucrose	Beet sugar Brown sugar Cane sugar Confectioner's sugar Invert sugar Powdered sugar Raw sugar Table sugar Turbinado	50% glucose. 50% fructose.
Sugar Alcohol	Dulcitol Mannitol Sorbitol Xylitol Hydrogenated starch hydrolysate	Not as sweet as sucrose. May cause diarrhea.
Syrups	Corn syrup Corn syrup solids and/or fructose High fructose syrups Honey maple syrup Molasses Sugar cane sugar Sorghum syrup	Primarily glucose.

Other Options for Sweetening Food

One simple way to keep "sweetness" in your meals without risking high blood sugar is to cut back on the amount of sugar used. With most recipes, you can reduce the sugar by at least one third without changing the taste and texture. For example, if the recipe calls for 1 cup of sugar, use ⅔ cup instead, and next time try ½ cup. Aim for a recipe that contains no more than 1 teaspoon of sugar per serving (1 cup of sugar = 48 teaspoons).

Another way to keep sweetness in your meals is to realize that many fresh fruits also taste sweet because they contain natural sugars. This makes fruit a good "sweet" choice.

Artificial, or Nonnutritive, Sweeteners

You also can reduce your carbohydrate intake from sugar by using artificial sweeteners. For example, aspartame (Equal or Nutrasweet) can be used in recipes that will be baked for less than 20 minutes, such as cookies or no-bake frozen desserts. Long exposure to heat causes aspartame to lose its sweetening power, so don't try this method in a long-baked dessert like apple pie. There are sweeteners that can be used in cooking and baking—saccharin (Sweet Magic, Sweet 'N Low, Sugar Twin) and acesulfame-K (Sweet One).

You cannot totally substitute artificial sweeteners for sugar in cakes or sweet breads. Why? Because the sugar provides bulk as well as sweetness to these recipes. Instead, try using a combination of sugar and a substitute. Cut the amount of sugar and use a substitute. Cut the amount of sugar by about ⅓ or ½, then replace the removed sugar with an artificial sweetener.

The following chart will help you calculate the correct amounts of sugar substitutes to use. Over time, it's better to use a little of each type of substitute, rather than a lot of one, thereby limiting the quantity of any one type you consume.

GUIDE FOR USING SUGAR SUBSTITUTES IN PLACE OF SUGAR

SUGAR	EQUAL (ASPARTAME)	SWEET 'N LOW (SACCHARIN)	SWEET ONE (ACESULFAME-K)
2 tsp	1 packet	⅕ tsp	1 packet
1 tbsp	1½ packets	⅓ tsp	1¼ packets
¼ cup	6 packets	3 packets	3 packets
⅓ cup	8 packets	4 packets	4 packets
½ cup	12 packets	6 packets (1 tbsp)	6 packets
⅔ cup	16 packets	8 packets	8 packets
¾ cup	18 packets	9 packets	9 packets
1 cup	24 packets	12 packets (2 tbsp)	12 packets

Here's another idea to add "sweetness" to your recipes. Use nutmeg, cinnamon, vanilla, or almond extract in place of some of the sugar. These flavorings give foods a sweet taste without adding sugar or calories.

"Dietetic" Foods

Such foods are often labeled "low calorie" or "reduced calorie." The label also states the number of calories per serving. (See Figure 4-1 for a typical product label and pages 62–68 for instructions on label reading.) Some of these foods may be helpful in adding flavor and variety to your meal plan. But try to limit their use to no more than 20 calories per serving in addition to the foods on your meal plan, and only consume them 2 to 3 times per day.

Don't confuse products labeled "dietetic" with "diabetic." The word *dietetic* simply means a product has been altered in some way. Perhaps an ingredient has been modified or omitted. It does not necessarily mean a product is low in calories. For example, a box of cookies marked dietetic may refer to the fact they are sodium-free, but they may contain large amounts of sugar. Or the manufacturer may have removed the table sugar (sucrose) but replaced it with another carbohydrate such as sorbitol, which provides the same number of calories as sugar. Read the labels carefully on dietetic foods. Consult with your dietitian if you are unsure about the use of any product.

Low-Calorie Foods
(*use in limited quantities*)

Diet jellies and jams (usually found in the dietetic section of stores)
Fruit jellies and jams such as Smuckers Low Sugar or Polaner's
All Fruit jellies and jams (usually found near the "regular" jellies and jams)
Diet syrups such as Cary's, DiaMel, or Featherweight
Sugar-free gelatin, such as Jell-O or D'Zerta brands
Sugar-free hard candy
Sugar-free gum

Sodium

Just as you have to watch your use of the sugar bowl at meals, so too do you need to watch how much you use the salt shaker. Most of the sodium we eat comes from *sodium chloride* (table salt) added to processed foods or sprinkled on foods during preparation or eating. Sodium also occurs naturally in a wide variety of foods.

Sodium is not a nutrient—it is a mineral. As such, it contains no molecules that can be converted into energy. However, certain minerals such as sodium are necessary for the proper functioning of your body. For example, sodium helps regulate the water balance in your body. It also plays a role in maintaining blood pressure.

Most Americans eat far more sodium than they need. Research also shows that sodium may contribute to some types of high blood pressure (*hypertension*), a problem that people with diabetes tend to have. Although not all people with diabetes have high blood pressure and not all high blood pressure is aggravated by sodium, it is recommended that people with diabetes limit their daily intake of sodium to 2,400 milligrams. By lowering your sodium intake, you may reduce your chances of aggravating high blood pressure and the risk of heart and blood-vessel disease.

Ways to Reduce Sodium

- Use salt sparingly during cooking or at the table. Always taste your food before adding salt.
- Rely less on canned, packaged, and convenience foods. Such foods tend to contain more sodium.
- Switch to low-sodium snacks. Instead of salted potato chips, nuts, and crackers, eat raw vegetables, unsalted crackers, and fruits.
- Use low-sodium flavor enhancers. Instead of salt, mustard, catsup, sauces, and other salt-filled flavorings, use herbs and spices, onion, green pepper, lemon juice, and vinegar.
- Eat fewer smoked or cured meats such as bacon, hot dogs, and cold cuts. Instead, select chicken, sliced turkey, and lean roast beef.
- Read food labels, which clearly state how much sodium is in foods.

Vitamins and Minerals

Last, but certainly not least, let's focus on vitamins and minerals such as calcium, iron, potassium, and zinc. These substances need to be present—but only in small amounts—in the foods we eat. They are very important because they help the body process foods and are involved in many other body functions.

People with diabetes often ask if they should take vitamin and mineral supplements, that is, capsules or tablets available from drugstores or health food stores. If you are eating a balanced diet—the whole idea behind a meal plan—you probably do not need to take these supplements.

However, recent medical studies have shown that certain vitamins, particularly vitamins C and E, may help prevent some of the long-term complications of diabetes, such as eye cataracts, retinopathy, nerve disorders, and blood-vessel disease. In some people, other medical conditions or treatments may affect their mineral balance which, in turn, will affect their diabetes. Ask your doctor if you are one of those people.

The bottom line is: If you wish to take vitamin and mineral supplements, be sure to check with your health-care team. Some of these substances can be toxic in large amounts, so it's important that you take only the recommended dose.

LABEL READING

If you look on the packaging of most foods in your grocery store, you will find detailed information about nutrition. Thanks to new federal food label regulations, this information clearly states how much carbohydrate, sodium, cholesterol, and fat a product contains. You then can decide whether it is appropriate for your use. In accordance with rulings by the Food and Drug Administration, labels on all U.S. products must state the "Nutrition Facts." You will find the calorie content of the product, and how many of the calories come from fat. They must also list the amounts of saturated fat, cholesterol, sodium, total carbohydrates (including sugars and dietary fiber), and protein. The vitamin and mineral content is also listed for vitamins A and C as well as the calcium and iron content.

Figure 4-1 is a typical product label. Let's go through it item by item to see how you can determine if a product is appropriate for your meal plan. But if after reading a label, you are still not sure, refer to the Food Choice Lists in the Appendix or consult with your dietitian.

Serving Size

The serving size listed on the package may be much less or more than you would normally eat. So you first need to determine how much of the product is a single serving for you because the nutritional information on the label is keyed directly to the serving size. If you are accustomed to eating more than what is called one serving, you must account for the extra amount. If you use the product, your best bet is to stick to the portion size on the food list given to you by your dietitian.

Nutrition Facts

Serving Size ½ cup (114 g)
Servings Per Container 4

Amount Per Serving

Calories 260	Calories From Fat 120

	% Daily Value*
Total Fat 13 g	20%
Saturated Fat 5 g	25%
Cholesterol 30 mg	10%
Sodium 660 mg	28%
Total Carbohydrate 31 g	10%
Dietary Fiber 0 g	0%
Sugars 5 g	
Protein 5 g	

Vitamin A 4%	•	Vitamin C 2%
Calcium 15%	•	Iron 4%

*Percent Daily Values are based on a 2,000 calorie diet. Your daily values may be higher or lower depending on your calorie needs:

	Calories:	2,000	2,500
Total Fat	Less than	65 g	80 g
Sat Fat	Less than	20 g	25 g
Cholesterol	Less than	300 mg	300 mg
Sodium	Less than	2,400 mg	2,400 mg
Total Carbohydrate		300 g	375 g
Dietary Fiber		25 g	30 g

Calories per gram:
Fat 9   •   Carbohydrate 4   •   Protein 4

Figure 4-1

Carbohydrates

Now with the recommendations for sugar somewhat relaxed in meal planning for people with diabetes, and the implementation of the label law of 1994, the *total* amount of carbohydrates should be the focus of your search when reading the label rather than the order of ingredients listed. Underneath "total carbohydrates" on the food label is listed the amount of "sugars" and the amount of "dietary fiber." Again, while people with diabetes for years have focused on that word "sugar," in fact it is the total carbohydrates that matter.

Types of Fat

It's best to choose products made from monounsaturated fats or polyunsaturated fats; that is, fats that come from nonanimal products such as vegetable oils. Choose items that list olive, canola, corn, and safflower oil. These fats tend to increase the amount of "good" cholesterol circulating in your blood without increasing the amount of "bad" cholesterol.

Avoid products that list saturated fats such as beef fat, lard, butter fat, coconut oil, or palm oil. Use caution for ingredients called "partially hydrogenated oils." These originally may have been unsaturated, but in processing, they have been made more saturated. When considering processed or convenience food products containing fat, try to choose those that you can fit into your eating plan.

Sodium per Serving

Sodium is listed as milligrams (mg) per serving on food labels. If you are considering keeping your sodium level down, try to choose foods that have less than 400 mg for a single serving or less than 800 mg for a convenience food or entrée.

Ranking of Ingredients

The nutritional ingredients of a food product are listed in descending order by weight. Listed first is the ingredient present in the largest amount by weight; the last ingredient is present in the smallest amount. If you use exchange meal planning, you can use this information to determine how to fit this product into your meal plan. More on this below.

PREPARED FOODS

Every grocery store is stocked with a wide assortment of prepared foods, ready-made entrees and dinners. Can you eat them? In many cases, yes. The directions below will help you learn how to fit various prepared foods into your meal plan.

To determine if a particular prepared food is suitable for your meal plan, you have to calculate how many "choices" from the various food groups a serving of the product provides. To do this, you should read the package label and compare the product nutrients with the Food Choice Lists (see Appendix).

A typical example of a label containing the nutritional content of a prepared food product appears below. To fit this or other products into your meal plan, follow this three-step procedure:

HEALTHY EDDIE'S CHICKEN AND PASTA DIVAN DINNER

Nutrition information	Per serving
Serving size	11.5 ounces
Servings per container	1
Calories	310
Protein	23 grams
Carbohydrate	45 grams
Fat	4 grams

Ingredients (partial listing): chicken breast meat, carrots, cooked vegetable rotini noodles, reconstituted dried sweet cream, apples . . .

STEP 1. Identify the major ingredients on the label. The major ingredients are listed first (generally the first four or five items), followed by items present in smaller amounts. The major ingredients in this product are chicken breast, carrots, noodles, reconstituted cream, and apples.

STEP 2. Determine the food group to which each major ingredient belongs. In this example, the major ingredients and the food groups to which they belong are:

Chicken breast	Meat group
Carrots	Vegetable group
Cooked vegetable rotini noodles	Bread/starch group
Reconstituted dried sweet cream	Fat group
Apples	Fruit group

STEP 3. The following table shows the grams of carbohydrate, protein, and fat in one choice from the various food groups. We'll use it in our calculations.

FOOD GROUP (ONE CHOICE)	CARBOHYDRATE (GRAMS)	PROTEIN (GRAMS)	FAT (GRAMS)
Milk			
Nonfat (skim)	12	8	0
Low-fat (1%)	12	8	3
Low-fat (2%)	12	8	5
Whole milk	12	8	8
Vegetable	5	2	0
Fruit	15	0	0
Bread	15	3	trace
Meat			
No-fat	0	7	0
Low-fat	0	7	3
Medium-fat	0	7	5
High-fat	0	7	8
Fat	0	0	5

To determine how many choices from each food group are provided by one serving of the product, compare the foregoing table to the ingredients found on the label as follows:

1. List the grams of carbohydrate, protein, and fat present in one serving of the product. For this example:

	CARBOHYDRATE	PROTEIN	FAT
Product	45 grams	23 grams	4 grams

2. Examine the grams of carbohydrate, protein, and fat present in one serving of the product. Notice that 45 grams of carbohydrate in the product equal the 45 grams in three bread choices in the food-group table above. Subtract the grams of carbohydrate, protein, and fat present in three bread choices from the number of these nutrients in one serving of the product.

	CARBOHYDRATE	PROTEIN	FAT
Product	45	23	4
Three bread choices	−45	−9	−0
Remainder	0	14	4

You have determined that one serving of the product provides three bread choices, plus some additional food choices.

3. Now notice that the remaining 14 grams of protein and 4 grams of fat are almost equal to two low-fat meat choices (1 low-fat meat

choice equals 7 grams of protein and 3 grams of fat). Subtract two meat choices from the product.

	CARBOHYDRATE	PROTEIN	FAT
Product	0	14	4
Two meat choices	− 0	− 14	− 6
Remainder	0	0	− 2

The result: You have determined that each serving provides three bread choices and two meat choices. The 2-gram difference between nutrients provided by the product and those included in the food choice is considered insignificant. As a rule of thumb, differences of 2 grams or less don't need to be counted.

Label Terms

The U.S. Department of Agriculture (USDA) regulates labels on most meat and poultry products. The Food and Drug Administration (FDA) regulates dairy products, fresh produce, seafood, and most processed foods. These agencies determine the way certain terms can be used on food products.

Manufacturers make a wide range of claims on their labels. For example, do you know the difference between *low calorie* and *low fat*? Use the glossary that follows to help you sort out foods that will lead to the healthiest eating.

Effective May 1994, the U.S. Food and Drug Administration requires the label terms listed below to have the following meanings:

Low fat

—For individual foods, "low fat" means no more than 3 grams of fat per serving.
—For main meals, "low fat" means no more than 30% of calories from fat.

Low in saturated fat

—No more than 1 gram of saturated fat per serving.
—No more than 15% of total calories from saturated fat.

Low sodium

—140 mg or less per serving.

Light, Lite

—One-third fewer calories or 50% less fat per serving.

—With respect to sodium, "light" can mean half the usual sodium content or less, but the label must state "light in sodium."

Low cholesterol

—For individual foods, no more than 20 mg of cholesterol and 2 g or less saturated fat per serving.

Reduced/less

—Means that a food contains 25% less of a nutrient than a comparable food.

Percent fat-free

—Can only be used on foods that are low-fat or fat-free to begin with.

DEVELOPING AN EATING STYLE

Your eating style—what, when, where, and why you eat—is very personal. It has developed from a variety of tastes and experiences during your lifetime. It is also affected by the stresses of everyday life: for example, caring for a family, a demanding job, and long commutes to work. Eating habits are acquired over many years and can be difficult to change—even if you need to because you have diabetes. However, with new understanding, you can learn many healthy eating habits. You can reorganize your schedule and develop a more healthful eating style.

The key to success is examining your current eating style and making appropriate changes. Begin by keeping a food diary for at least one week. Record WHAT, WHEN, WHERE, and WHY you ate. "What" you eat is fairly straightforward. Be sure to record everything. "When" and "where" are also important, especially if your notes reveal a pattern of times and places that you tend to overeat. Do you eat more if you are watching TV? While standing in front of the refrigerator? In bed? "Why" also is important. Are you really hungry, or do you eat because you are bored or depressed? When you have these feelings, try to find other activities to substitute for eating.

Ask your family and friends for support with your eating style. If you tend to overeat when preparing foods, perhaps others could cook for you. If you are trying to lose weight, ask someone to encourage you. Keep high-fat foods that other family members may buy in places hard to reach. Or keep them out of the house entirely. Make it easy to eat what you should. For example, place a bowl of fruit on the kitchen table.

Expect your eating habits to change slowly. They have developed over time and are difficult to modify quickly. Ask your health-care team for help. Your dietitian can provide new ways to prepare food, new recipes, and encouragement. Using home blood glucose monitoring results, you can learn how to incorporate foods you previously thought you couldn't eat into your meals. Remember, you are not trying to follow a short-term diet. You are developing a lifelong eating style that will help you properly manage your diabetes and will also benefit your overall health.

CHAPTER 5

The Exercise Prescription

YOUR BODY IS MADE for movement—arms that bend, legs that run, and a heart that beats every second of the day. It only makes sense that if something is designed for movement, it's good practice to move it regularly! Indeed, exercise is good for everyone. It helps tone and strengthen muscles. It also gives your heart and lungs a workout, helping them work more efficiently and providing you with more energy.

WHY YOU NEED EXERCISE

Regular exercise is especially good for people with diabetes. It provides benefits that you will realize daily as well as throughout your life. On a daily basis, exercise can help you maintain your blood sugar within a normal range. Almost immediately, regular activity will make your body's cells more sensitive to insulin, which makes it more effective, allowing people with diabetes to use less medication. In fact, research suggests that exercise can actually help prevent Type II diabetes. People who are at risk for this kind of diabetes—people who are overweight, over age 40, or have a family history of diabetes—would be well advised to make exercise a top priority.

How else does regular exercise benefit you? It can help lower the levels of "bad" (LDL) cholesterol and triglycerides in the blood. If you have too much of these blood fats, you are more likely to develop blood-vessel disease (*atherosclerosis*). In this disease, fatty deposits settle in your arteries and clog them. The condition is especially serious when buildup occurs in the vessels that supply the heart and brain. Eventually, the arteries of these vital organs may close down, causing a heart attack or stroke.

Exercise also increases the level of "good" (HDL) cholesterol. This type of cholesterol "sweeps" the fatty deposits from the arteries, protecting you from blood-vessel disease. People with diabetes have a greater tendency to develop this problem. That's why it's so important to lower your blood cholesterol through nutrition and exercise.

Finally, if you are overweight, a regular exercise program can go a long way toward helping you lose extra pounds. Teamed with a good meal plan, exercise can help you get down to a desired weight and maintain that weight. The result is that you look better and feel better. And your diabetes is much easier to control.

How Exercise Affects Blood Sugars

Exercise, diet, and medication are part of a delicate balancing act, all working together to keep your blood sugar in a normal range. It's important to know how exercise affects your blood sugar. That way, you'll have a better idea of how to adjust food and medication around the time you exercise.

Exercise involves muscles, particularly the large skeletal muscles of your arms and legs. Muscles generally use two fuels—glucose (blood sugar) and fatty acids—to get the energy they need to work. Here's how the body normally burns fuel during exercise:

Phase 1. During the first short bursts of activity, the muscles in the body use their own sugar first.

Phase 2. As you continue exercising, the body uses sugar stored in the liver, which is transported through the bloodstream to the muscles. This replenishes the blood sugar.

Phase 3. After about 30–40 minutes, the body begins to burn body fat in the form of fatty acids for fuel.

Insulin plays a key role in exercise because it enables the body to use blood sugar for energy. Besides insulin, other hormones get into the act during exercise. These hormones tell the liver to produce more or less glucose, as needed. They also trigger the breakdown of fat tissue into fatty acids.

Low Insulin

What happens if there is *not enough* insulin circulating in the blood during exercise? Without enough insulin, glucose can't get into the cells to provide them with energy and so it begins to back up in the bloodstream. The liver senses that the cells are "starved" for glucose and mistakenly begins to make *more* glucose, pumping it into the bloodstream. But there wasn't enough insulin to take care of the glucose in the first place. Now there's even more! The result: The muscles don't get any glucose, and the level of blood sugar climbs higher and higher.

High Insulin

Now let's look at the flip side of the coin. What if there's *too much* insulin in the blood during exercise? Sensing the high level of insulin, the liver mistakenly assumes there is plenty of glucose available, so it slows its production of glucose. At the same time, the muscles increase their use of glucose. The result: The level of blood sugar falls quickly, sometimes causing low blood sugar (*hypoglycemia*).

When to Exercise

For all the above reasons, DO NOT begin an exercise program if your blood sugar levels are above 240 mg/dl without first testing your urine for ketones (see Chapter 10 for information on how to test for ketones). These substances are produced when the body starts to burn fatty acids. If ketones are present, do not exercise until the source of the problem has been found and corrected. If your blood sugar level is over 240 mg/dl, but *no ketones* are present, follow the guidelines below, depending on your type of diabetes.

- *Type I*—Do not exercise if your blood sugar is 300 mg/dl or higher.
- *Children with Type I*—Do not exercise if your blood sugar is 400 mg/dl or higher.
- *Type II*—Regardless of whether or not you use insulin, do not exercise when your blood sugar is 400 mg/dl or higher.

CREATING YOUR EXERCISE PROGRAM

What makes a good exercise program? Actually, there is no single program that is right for every person with diabetes. You need to develop a program based on your lifestyle, interests, and physical abilities. This can be done by consulting with a specialist called an *exercise physiologist*. This person is a member of your diabetes health-care team and is trained in how the body responds to exercise. Together, you can create a program that fits your medical needs and lifestyle.

In designing your exercise program, you and your exercise physiologist will be following some general guidelines for people with diabetes.

Consult Your Physician

Before beginning a new exercise program, consult your physician about your overall physical condition. Getting your doctor's approval is important, whether you have diabetes or not, but it's especially important for people with diabetes. It's an absolute "must" if you are over age 35 or if you have had diabetes for 20 years or more. That's because some forms of exercise can actually be dangerous for people with certain complications from diabetes. For example, diabetic eye disease can be made worse by exercise that involves a lot of bouncing and impact. People with diabetes must also be careful about their feet if they have nerve damage (neuropathy) or circulation problems. And if they have heart disease, they must avoid exercise that puts strain on the heart.

Make Sure Your Diabetes Is Under Control

Before starting your exercise program, be certain your diabetes is adequately controlled and you know what adjustments to make in your diabetes program for the increased activity. If you start a new program when your diabetes is not properly controlled, it can lead to serious problems such as *ketoacidosis*. This condition occurs when the blood becomes too *acidic* due to the buildup of ketones, and it can result in coma and even death.

Choose the Right Form of Exercise

The best exercise for a person with diabetes is a continuous activity that uses large amounts of energy over a period of time—about 20 to 40 minutes without interruption. Examples of such exercise include brisk walking, running, jogging, bicycling, tennis, cross-country skiing, racquetball, swimming, and jumping rope. These activities help maintain good blood sugar control. Some forms of exercise are less helpful in managing blood sugar. Stop-and-go activities such as bowling, softball, and some calisthenics use only short bursts of energy. If you need some advice in picking a suitable activity, ask your physician or exercise physiologist. Again, be aware that depending on your condition, there may be forms of exercise that you should avoid.

Choose Activities You Enjoy

Exercise is easier if you're doing something you like. If you pick something grueling, you might soon become an "exercise dropout." Fortunately, there are many activities that help people with diabetes maintain good blood control, as shown in Table 5-1. In choosing a form of exercise, consider whether the necessary equipment and facilities are convenient to your home or workplace. If not, you may become discouraged and abandon your program. Walking is one of the best forms of exercise—and you can walk almost anywhere!

TABLE 5-1. PHYSICAL ACTIVITIES FOR PEOPLE WITH DIABETES

Individual Activities

Brisk walking	Running or jogging
Swimming	Bicycling (including stationary)
Dancing	Skipping rope
Rowing	Skiing (downhill and cross-country)
Badminton	Skating (ice and roller)
Wrestling	Golf (with brisk walking only!)
Fencing	Stair climbing
Calisthenics	Tennis
Handball	Squash
Racquetball	

Team Activities

Soccer	Volleyball (vigorous only!)
Basketball	Hockey (ice and field)
Lacrosse	

Other Activities, If Done at the Proper Intensity

Digging	Wood cutting and splitting
Lawn mowing	Farming

Exercise Regularly

Exercising every day is best. But if you can't do that, plan to exercise at least every other day (3 to 4 times a week). This is essential to help keep your blood sugar in control. If you have trouble finding a time for exercise, look at your daily schedule and identify days and times that you can reserve for exercise—perhaps before or after work or during your lunch break. To stay true to your schedule, make a chart and post it in a conspicuous place—next to the back door or on your bathroom mirror.

Identify the Best Time for Exercise

You'll get the most out of your program if you exercise at the most appropriate time. Exercise helps lower your blood sugar. For that reason, it is very important to choose the best time for exercise. If you don't, you may have to eat more food to keep your blood sugar from dropping too low, and that could have an impact on your weight-control program.

In general, the best time to exercise is about an hour after meals, when your blood sugar level is the highest, so your risks of hypoglycemia (low blood sugar) are lowest. Also, you're more likely to lose weight because you won't have to eat extra food to ward off low blood sugar. Moreover, it's not a good idea to exercise when your diabetes pills or insulin injections are working at their peak activity. This could also cause low blood sugar.

Test Your Blood Sugar

For the first three weeks of an exercise program, it's a good idea to test blood sugar four times a day—before each meal and at bedtime. If you use insulin, you should also test your blood sugar before every exercise session and take note of the last time you ate. *Everyone* with diabetes should check his or her blood sugar immediately after exercising, or at least within 15 minutes. That way, you'll spot any problems you may be having in controlling your blood sugar.

Respond to Low or High Blood Sugar

If you use insulin, your blood sugar after exercise should be between 100 and 120 mg/dl. If you use diabetes pills or take no medication to manage your diabetes, your blood sugar level should be no lower than 80 mg/dl. If your blood sugar falls outside the normal range from exercise, there are measures you can take to bring it under control. The two major types of adjustments—through food and medication—are discussed in greater detail later in this chapter.

Ease into Your Program

Don't dive into a full-scale exercise program. If you haven't been very active, begin with a brief period of exercise. Recent research shows that doing even small amounts of exercise is better than doing nothing at all. To ease into your program, you may want to try walking 10 to 20 minutes a day, then build up to 30 or 45 minutes each day over a span of several weeks. Always begin with a warm-up and finish with a cool-down.

Table 5-2 can help you determine how often and how long you should exercise each week. First, look at the left-hand column to choose the activity level that best describes your present situation. Move to the second column to learn how often you should exercise. The third column identifies the length of time you should exercise during each session, and the fourth how much time per week. The fifth column identifies the intensity of the exercise—i.e., the heart rate you should achieve during exercise.

TABLE 5-2. THE EXERCISE PRESCRIPTION

This table lists the various levels of activity by frequency, duration, time, and intensity. Unless you are currently more active than the "sedentary" level, you should start at that level and work your way up.

ACTIVITY LEVEL	FREQUENCY (SESSIONS PER WEEK)	DURATION (MINUTES PER SESSION)	TOTAL TIME PER WEEK (MINUTES)	INTENSITY (HEART RATE DURING EXERCISE)
Sedentary	4–6	10–20	40–80	100–120
Somewhat active	4–6	15–30	90–120	100–130
Moderately active	3–5	30–45	120–180	110–140
Very active	3–5	30–60	180–300	120–160
Athlete	5–7	60–120	300–840	140–190

Exercise Your Heart

Exercise not only helps you manage your diabetes, but also contributes to the fitness of your heart. But this can happen only if the exercise is sufficiently intense. For exercise to be of value, your heart rate must rise to a certain number of beats per minute and remain there during the activity period. Your heart rate should be between 60 and 85 percent of your maximum heartbeat rate. If you are just beginning, stay toward the low end of your target heart rate—that is, more toward the 60 percent level.

Here's how to compute the heart rate you should achieve during exercise if you don't have high blood pressure, heart problems, or diabetes complications. (If you do, consult your exercise physiologist or doctor.) First, determine your maximum heart rate by subtracting your age from the number 220. For example, if you are 35 years old, your maximum heart rate is 220 minus 35, or 185. Now take 60 and 85 percent of 185 (0.60 × 185 = 111; 0.85 × 185 = 157). The rate you should achieve during exercise is 111 to 157 heartbeats per minute.

Table 5-3 lists average maximum heart rates for people of various ages and the heart rates they should achieve during exercise. You can use the chart as a general guideline to determine your safe heart rate during exercise.

TABLE 5-3

AGE	AVERAGE MAXIMUM HEART RATE	HEART RATE TO ACHIEVE DURING EXERCISE*
20 years	200	120–170
25 years	195	117–166
30 years	190	114–162
35 years	185	111–157
40 years	180	108–153
45 years	175	105–149
50 years	170	102–145
55 years	165	99–140
60 years	160	96–136
65 years	155	93–132
70 years	150	90–128

* You can check your heartbeat rate while exercising by placing the tip of a finger on the pulse on the thumb side of your wrist or on the side of your neck and counting the beats for 10 seconds. Multiply the number of beats by 6 to obtain the number of beats per minute.

Develop a Routine

Your exercise physiologist can help you create a good routine. An effective exercise program should consist of the following phases:

- *Warm-up phase*—5 to 10 minutes at a slower pace, increasing the speed gradually.
- *Cardiovascular phase*—your pace is brisker and your breathing may increase for 20 to 30 minutes.

• *Cool-down phase*—final 5 to 10 minutes in which you gradually slow your pace and return to a resting state.

Table 5-4 is a sample exercise session that involves all these phases.

TABLE 5-4. WALKING FOR EXERCISE

Warm-up: For the first 5 to 10 minutes, walk slowly, perhaps slightly faster than the pace you normally walk.

Cardiovascular: During the next 30 minutes, build up your speed to a brisk rate. Halfway through this period, your pace should be at its highest point. Take your pulse rate at this time. If it is under or over your target heart rate, speed up or slow down for the rest of this phase (the next 15 minutes).

Cool-down: Gradually begin walking more slowly over the next 5 to 10 minutes. At the end, do some arm and leg stretches.

GUIDELINES AND PRECAUTIONS

Exercise can do your body a tremendous amount of good. But when you have diabetes, you should be prepared to respond to low blood sugar or other reactions to exercise. If you experience low blood sugar after exercise, there are two primary ways to adjust your treatment program—through changes in food and medication.

Adjusting Food

During physical activity, your muscles use much more sugar for energy than when your body is at rest. This can cause your blood sugar to fall rapidly. Therefore, you must be careful to maintain blood sugar within a satisfactory range while exercising.

To do this, you must balance:

1. The sugar needed for energy while exercising
2. The sugar available from food
3. And the action pattern of your injected insulin, if you use insulin

Sometimes, you may need extra food to maintain this balance during exercise. Making food adjustments will depend on a number of factors. Table 5-5 lists some guidelines for making these adjustments. These guidelines are general because your food requirements will depend on

TABLE 5-5

TYPE OF EXERCISE AND EXAMPLES	IF BLOOD GLUCOSE IS	SUGGESTIONS OF FOOD TO USE
Exercise of short duration (30 minutes or less) and of moderate intensity Examples: walking a mile or bicycling for less than 30 minutes	Less than 100 100–180 180 or more	1 fruit + 1 bread + 1 meat 1 bread or 1 fruit Snack *may* not be necessary
Exercise of intermediate duration (1 hour) and moderate intensity Examples: tennis, swimming, jogging, leisurely bicycling, gardening, golfing, or vacuuming for one hour	Less than 100 100–180 180–240 240 or more	1 fruit + 1 bread + 1 meat 1 bread + 1 meat 1 bread or 1 fruit Snack *may* not be necessary
Exercise of long duration (2 hours or more) and high intensity Examples: football, hockey, racquetball or basketball games; strenuous bicycling or swimming; shoveling heavy snow, skiing, hiking	Consult with your physician or exercise physiologist. Insulin may need to be decreased by 30%–75%. Begin with a snack of 2 bread + 2 meat and then eat at least 1 bread or 1 fruit per hour of exercise. Test hourly. If blood glucose is 180 or more, an extra snack *may* not be needed for that hour.	

the activity you choose. Therefore, use the guidelines only as a starting point. Over time, trial and error will help you determine if you need to make adjustments. Be sure to ask your exercise physiologist for help.

Monitoring your blood sugar (discussed in Chapter 10) will give you important information about how exercise is affecting your blood sugar. Be sure to test your blood sugar before and after exercising. You may also want to test while exercising. Keep good written monitoring records which include your blood sugar level, insulin dose, food consumption, and exercise, so that you can learn from your experience.

To determine if you need extra food while exercising, you should consider these factors:

- The time your medication is working
- Whether or not you have just eaten a meal
- The duration and intensity of the activity
- The results from monitoring your blood sugar

Depending on your particular situation, you may need to eat before, during, or after exercise. Good rules of thumb:

- If the exercise is planned, you can decrease the medication that is active at the time of exercise.
- If the exercise is unplanned, you should increase your food.
- If weight loss is your goal, you should always plan your exercise, thereby limiting the amount of extra food you need to keep your blood sugar from dropping too low. Exercising 1 to 2 hours after meals is often the best time.

Adjust Your Medication

Another way to get blood sugar under control during exercise is to adjust medication. But before adjusting your medication, always seek the advice of your health-care team. If you use pills to treat your diabetes, your doctor may suggest that you use less medication to keep your blood sugar from going too low during exercise. If you use insulin, you may be advised to reduce the dose of insulin that is active at the time you exercise. For example, your doctor and exercise physiologist may suggest reducing that dose by 10 percent (one-tenth).

Table 5-6 shows several ways to adjust insulin for exercise. The adjustment will depend on the intensity of the exercise, how long it lasts, and the type of insulin that is acting during exercise. For example, you may take short-acting "regular" insulin in the morning and plan to exercise after breakfast, which is when the insulin is acting. If you were taking 10 units of regular insulin, you would reduce your dose by 1 unit ($0.10 \times 10 = 1$). Your new morning dose would be 9 units. Test your blood sugar after exercise to make sure your adjustments are accurate.

Special Precautions

1. **Exercising before meals.** While it's best to exercise about 1 to 2 hours *after* a meal, sometimes you may find yourself exercising *before* meals. When you exercise immediately before a meal, you need to take precautions to prevent low blood sugar. Blood sugar levels are usually

TABLE 5-6. INSULIN ADJUSTMENT GUIDELINES FOR EXERCISE

% TO DECREASE PEAKING INSULIN	INTENSITY OF EXERCISE	DURATION OF EXERCISE
0%	Low, moderate, or high intensity	Short duration
5%	Low intensity	Intermediate to long duration
10%	Moderate intensity	Intermediate duration
20%	Moderate intensity	Long duration
20%	High intensity	Intermediate duration
30%	High intensity	Long duration

Duration of Exercise:

Short = less than 30 minutes (not necessary to adjust insulin)
Intermediate = 30–60 minutes
Long = 60 minutes or more

Intensity of Exercise:

High intensity = high end of target heart rate
Moderate intensity = low end of target heart rate
Low intensity = not in target zone

Adjust the Insulin Acting During the Exercise Time:

Regular insulin peak action	2 to 4 hours
NPH/Lente insulin peak action	6 to 12 hours
Ultralente insulin peak action	18 to 24 hours
(Do not adjust Ultralente insulin)	

lowest before meals, and exercise will lower them even further. Therefore, you may need to eat a snack before exercising.

If you exercise before a meal, test your blood sugar level before you begin. Use Table 5-5 to determine the amount and type of snack needed. It's important not to eat too large a snack because your blood sugar level might rise after exercise. Test your blood sugar immediately after your exercise period. This will help determine if you need a larger or smaller snack the next time you exercise.

An exception to the above procedure: If your blood sugar is high and you are trying to lower it through exercise, you may not need the extra snack.

2. Exercising when insulin action is peaking. If you exercise during periods of the day when your insulin is working hardest (peak time), special precautions should be taken. Otherwise, the combination of insulin action and exercise may cause blood sugar levels to fall below the normal range. For example, if you take a mixed dose of short- and intermediate-acting insulin at 7 A.M., it will peak at approximately 10 A.M. and again at 3 P.M. Exercising during these periods is more likely to cause your blood sugar to fall below normal.

If you exercise when your insulin is peaking, you should eat extra food before beginning the activity. Use Table 5-7 as a guideline. A snack containing 10–15 grams of carbohydrate would be appropriate for less than an hour of exercise. Add 7–8 grams of protein if you exercise one hour or more. Also, if you know the time of exercise in advance, you can reduce the dose of insulin peaking at that time by 10–20 percent, depending on the duration and intensity of the exercise.

3. *Preventing ketoacidosis.* Exercising when your blood sugar is consistently high, due to insufficient insulin, may cause it to rise even higher and lead to the formation of ketones. That may result in *keto-acidosis*, the life-threatening situation in which there is too much acid in the blood. *Do not* exercise when your blood sugar is greater than 300 mg/dl if you have Type I diabetes, or 400 mg/dl if you have Type II diabetes. (Children with Type I diabetes can exercise as long as their blood sugar levels are not over 400 mg/dl.) You should also avoid exercise when blood sugar is 240 mg/dl or more and ketones are present at the time of exercise. You need to bring your diabetes under satisfactory control before exercising.

4. *Avoiding low blood sugar after strenuous exercise.* Low blood sugar may occur 12 to 24 hours after a period of vigorous exercise. This is known as the "lag effect." An occasional problem for people who use insulin, it can occur a day or two after exercise. Why? Because during exercise, there is an increased demand for the stored glucose in your skeletal muscles and liver. After exercise, the body works to replenish these reserves, drawing on the sugar circulating in the blood, which can cause your blood sugar to plunge.

TABLE 5-7

FOODS CONTAINING 10–15 GRAM S OF CARBOHYDRATE (EQUALS 1 BREAD OR 1 FRUIT)	FOODS CONTAINING 7–8 GRAMS OF PROTEIN (EQUALS 1 MEAT)
Small piece of fresh fruit	1 ounce of low-fat cheese
2 tablespoons of raisins	¼ cup of low-fat cheese
5–7 dried apricot halves	1 ounce of poultry or lean meat
4–6 crackers	¼ cup of tuna or salmon
1 slice of bread	1 tablespoon of peanut butter

To avoid low blood sugar after a particularly strenuous and prolonged period of exercise, you should have an extra snack at the end of the activity. Be sure to test blood sugar levels at bedtime on days you engage in especially vigorous exercise. If your level of blood sugar is 100 mg/dl or less, take a double bedtime snack.

If you participate in an all-day activity such as hiking, cross-country skiing, canoeing, or biking, you may need a small snack every 30–60 minutes to prevent low blood sugar. Your total insulin dose should also be reduced by 20–30 percent. Consult your physician or exercise physiologist for guidance prior to such activities. Frequent testing of your blood sugar levels is essential during the activity.

5. *Determining the cause of high blood sugar after exercise.* If your blood sugar level is high 30 minutes after exercise, you should determine the cause. It may be due to a preexercise snack that was too large. Or if you exercised shortly after a meal, the high blood sugar may stem from the food you recently ate.

6. *Exercising for weight loss.* If you are exercising to help lose weight, monitor your blood sugar carefully after exercising and focus on decreasing your insulin dose instead of increasing food if you are experiencing low blood sugars. See guidelines for reducing insulin doses in Table 5-6.

7. *What to do on sick days.* If you are sick, don't exercise until your blood sugar is back to normal. Never exercise if your blood sugar levels are consistently above the guidelines listed on page 72 or if ketones are present.

8. *Safety considerations.* Do not exercise alone in isolated areas, especially if you are prone to insulin reactions (low blood sugar), which can result in unconsciousness. Exercise with a family member or friend.

9. *Carry identification.* Always carry some form of identification that says you have diabetes. The identification should include your name, address, phone number, physician's name and phone number, the type and dose of insulin and other medications you use. This will help other people know how to assist you if you get into difficulty.

10. *Be prepared for low blood sugar.* Sometimes low blood sugar occurs during exercise, despite your best efforts. Always be prepared for such a situation. Carry a concentrated form of carbohydrate, such as packets of granulated sugar, glucose tablets, cake icing, or LifeSavers. If your activities involve other people, tell them about the risk of low blood sugar and what they should do to help.

11. *Insulin absorption.* For many years, people were advised not to inject insulin in an arm or leg immediately before exercise. It was

believed that the pumping effect of muscles used during exercise would speed up the rate of insulin absorption from the injection site and cause the level of blood sugar to drop rapidly. By moving the site of injection to a nonworking muscle, an insulin reaction might be avoided. While it's now believed that the pumping effect of muscles during exercise has some effect on insulin absorption, simply moving the injection site will not likely prevent low blood sugar. To avoid low blood sugar, it is more important to pay close attention to the timing of your injection and the activity pattern of the insulin you are using. These will be discussed further in Chapter 8.

12. *Special guidelines for people who do not use insulin.* If you use diabetes pills to manage your blood sugar, you may need to adjust your medication to prevent low blood sugar following exercise. If your blood sugar falls below 80 mg/dl after physical activity, you will need to decrease your medication.

Also, test, test, test your blood sugar! Just because you do not use insulin does not mean you should avoid this important part of your care. Don't just eat a snack because you "feel" your blood sugar is low. Always check!

If you are trying to lose weight, it's important to plan the best time for exercise. That way, you can avoid eating extra food to counteract the low blood sugar that can occur if you exercise at the wrong time.

MAKING IT ALL WORTHWHILE

People with diabetes are often amazed at how well exercise can help control their blood sugar. Combined with meal planning and the appropriate medication, it is a vital part of your overall treatment program. And aside from the physical benefits, exercise can give you a big psychological boost. It causes your body to release chemicals called *endorphins*, which increase your sense of well-being. Exercise also can help you manage stress better and improve your self-image through weight loss. In short, exercise will help you control your diabetes and perhaps improve your entire outlook on life.

CHAPTER 6

Losing Weight— Gaining Control

YOUR BODY WORKS much like an orchestra. It's made up of "instrument sections," the major systems in your body that work in concert to keep you alive and well. The circulatory system, headed by the heart, pumps blood throughout your body. Along the way, the blood picks up nutrients broken down by the digestive system. Meanwhile the respiratory system, led by the lungs, supplies oxygen to the blood. There are many other bodily systems, all working in harmony. And the way you treat these systems will affect your overall health.

But like an orchestra, your body can get out of tune. And one of the harshest things you can do to your body is to be overweight. Carrying around extra pounds makes the heart work harder and less efficiently. You tire quickly and become short of breath. But most importantly for people with Type II diabetes, being overweight somehow affects your body's ability to use insulin. That's why your doctor may advise you to lose weight—to get your body as closely back "in tune" as possible.

The combination of a proper meal plan and exercise is the most effective way to lose weight. Simple adjustments to your thinking can also help change behaviors that may be preventing you from shedding unwanted pounds. But before you begin a weight-loss program, it's important to get an okay from your physician. Also plan to consult with your entire health-care team. They can help you develop a game plan based on sound medical principles.

WHY LOSE WEIGHT?

Many people with Type II diabetes are advised to lose weight. If you have this type of diabetes, your body still produces insulin. The main problem is that the insulin isn't working as well as it could. However, research has shown that when you are at a lower weight, more of the insulin receptors on your cells will be available than is the case at higher weights. Thus the insulin your body produces will be more effective in allowing blood sugar to pass into the cells, which results in lower blood sugar and gives you more energy.

There are other reasons to lose weight. Everyone can reduce the risk of heart and blood-vessel disease by following a low-fat diet and getting plenty of exercise. But if you have diabetes, you run a higher risk of developing these problems. That's why it's important to get on board with good nutrition and regular exercise.

Weight loss can even affect your use of insulin. If you have Type II diabetes, you may be taking insulin to help control your condition because your body isn't producing enough insulin to keep your blood sugar in the normal range. Diabetes pills may have worked for a time. But after many years, these medications may have lost their effectiveness. You may have been placed on insulin therapy. However, small amounts of weight loss can change your insulin needs significantly. By losing as little as 10 to 20 pounds, your blood sugar may come down. In fact, with enough weight loss, some people with Type II diabetes can actually stop using insulin or diabetes pills!

Because your insulin needs will probably change as you lose weight, plan to check your blood sugar daily, then discuss the results with your health-care team. They will adjust your insulin dose or show you how to adjust it. In making adjustments, keep in mind that insulin peaks in your body at certain times. Your meals and snacks should be planned to fit that pattern.

A TWO-PART EQUATION

The concept behind losing weight is rather simple. You need to burn up more calories than you eat. There are two basic ways to do that:

- Increase your activity—the reason for regular exercise
- Cut back on your food intake—the reason for your meal plan

What's the best way to set about losing weight? You've probably seen ads for many fad diets, and while they may claim dramatic results, the reality is that most of them don't work. Indeed, you might be able to shed 10 pounds quickly. But most people gain it all back, primarily because they haven't learned a lifelong eating style that will help them take weight off and keep it off. In fact, some weight-loss gimmicks are too extreme for most people to follow long enough to achieve true fat loss. Often they lose only a lot of body fluids, not body mass. Remember, you want to lose fat, not just water.

There's actually a dangerous aspect to some crash diets. They can deprive your body of nutrients that you need. If you have diabetes, this is a special concern. You need a balance of foods with specific nutrients to control your blood sugar. If you are taking insulin or diabetes pills to manage your diabetes, an imbalance of nutrients could lead to high blood sugar (*hyperglycemia*) or low blood sugar (*hypoglycemia*).

There's something else you should know about *any* diet. Reducing calories may slow your body's metabolism, the rate at which calories are burned. This makes it even harder to lose weight. However, regular exercise can help minimize this slowdown in metabolism. That's one of the reasons you should plan to make physical activity an important part of your program to lose weight.

MEAL PLANNING—HALF THE EQUATION

If you have diabetes, your health-care team has probably advised you to follow a meal plan. A well-designed meal plan can be an ideal way to achieve and maintain near normal blood sugar levels and lose weight. But it's more than a way to balance meals with medication, and it's more than a strategy to lose weight. Your meal plan is a blueprint for well-balanced nutrition.

If you're trying to shed extra pounds, your first goal is to get down to a reasonable body weight. We now believe that for some people it is physiologically impossible to achieve and maintain a "normal" body weight that makes them look like a movie star. If you are one of these people, the way you will be able to measure whether you have achieved an adequate and successful weight loss will not be by looking at your bathroom scale, but by looking at what your blood sugars are. A successful weight loss will be one that enables you to keep your blood sugars in a more normal range.

Table 6-1. Desirable Weight Ranges—Ages 25 and Over*

HEIGHT (NO SHOES) (FEET, INCHES)	MEN		WOMEN†	
	WEIGHT RANGE	AVG. WEIGHT‡ (POUNDS)	WEIGHT RANGE	AVG. WEIGHT‡ (POUNDS)
4 9			90–118	100
4 10			92–121	103
4 11			95–124	106
5 0			98–127	109
5 1	105–134	117	101–130	112
5 2	108–137	120	104–134	116
5 3	111–144	123	107–138	120
5 4	114–145	126	110–142	124
5 5	117–149	129	114–146	128
5 6	121–154	133	118–150	132
5 7	125–159	138	122–154	136
5 8	129–163	142	126–159	140
5 9	133–167	146	130–164	144
5 10	137–172	150	134–169	148
5 11	141–177	155		
6 0	145–182	159		
6 1	149–187	164		
6 2	153–192	169		
6 3	157–197	174		

* Adapted from the 1959 Metropolitan Desirable Weight Table (weight in pounds, without clothing; height without shoes). † For women between the ages of 18 and 25, subtract one pound for each year under 25. ‡ Average weight for person with medium frame

As you learn to modify your eating habits by using home blood glucose monitoring and boosting your activity, you can lose weight and achieve good blood sugar control. If you have diabetes, it is especially important to consult with the dietitian on your health-care team. With your dietitian's help, you'll learn the value of meal plans and the impact on your blood sugar level. You'll learn which foods to avoid and which foods are helpful in managing your diabetes. These topics are discussed in detail in Chapters 3 and 4 of this guide. But in general, if you are trying to lose weight, your dietitian will devise a meal plan based on a simple concept. Your total intake of calories should be less than what you now consume (to stay at your current weight).

Your weight-loss motto should be "slow and steady." The following formulas explain how to lose at a healthy rate—½ to 1 pound per week. Using these formulas, in half a year you will have shed up to 25 pounds.

One pound of body fat is equal to about 3,500 calories. Therefore, if you cut your food intake by 500 calories a day for seven days (500 × 7 = 3,500), you will lose approximately 1 pound of fat per week. Also, if you exercise and burn 250 extra calories a day for seven days (250 × 7 = 1,750), you will lose about half a pound a week.

Mind over Matter

A big part of winning the weight-loss battle is changing how you think about maintaining your weight. One way is to change the words you use:

- Rather than "losing weight," think of gaining the overall benefits that come from exercising every day and eating fewer high-fat foods.
- Instead of feeling "deprived" of food, think of enjoying more low-fat foods.
- Rather than the word "diet," use the term *meal plan*.

You may also have to change some behaviors that are standing in your way to success. No one can lose weight for you, and it's important that you *personally* accept the responsibility for managing your weight-loss program. It will be harder to follow a program if you shift the responsibility to other people or allow them to take it upon themselves. You should become directly involved in your meal-plan decisions, perhaps accompanying your spouse to the grocery store. You should take part in planning and preparing your meals and snacks. That doesn't mean your family has to stay completely out of the picture. In fact, they can give you a lot of support. So be sure to invite them to meetings with your health-care team when weight loss and eating plans are discussed.

Shifting the Balance

Everything that you eat can be classified into three main nutrient groups—carbohydrates, protein, and fat. All are important sources of calories. But because there are significant differences in the way these nutrients affect your blood sugar, a shift in their balance in your meal plan can help you lose weight. Remember, every gram of fat contains twice as many calories as carbohydrates and protein. If you are trying to lose weight, your meal plan may include a larger proportion of calories from carbohydrates than would a person's not trying to lose weight. You will eat less calories from fat. For ways to reduce fat and cholesterol in your meal plan, see Chapter 4.

Fat-Gram Counting

If you have Type II diabetes, you will be able to manage your diabetes better if you reduce the amount of fat tissue in your body while maintaining muscle. That's because muscle tissue has more receptor sites for the insulin your body is making. By cutting back on the amount of fat in your meals, you will be better able to lose unwanted body fat that may be interfering with your diabetes control. And there's another good reason to reduce dietary fat. Recent studies have shown that a high-fat diet can bring about obesity—even without eating an excess amount of calories!

One way to cut back on dietary fat is with a meal-planning technique called "fat-gram counting." With this method, your dietitian looks at your individual needs and determines the total amount of fat grams that you should eat in a day. On a daily basis, you then keep records of your fat intake. Using a "fat-gram counter," a chart that lists the number of grams of fat in different foods, you target the amount of fat in your present meal plan and reduce that amount by choosing foods that are lower in fat. Fat-gram counting will help you reduce your total fat intake to the goal set by your dietitian. If you're interested in this approach, however, be sure to first discuss it with the members of your health-care team. They will make sure that you're getting the proper nutrition while maintaining good control of your blood sugar.

High-Fiber Foods

Foods high in fiber are also good for a weight-loss program. That's because fiber has plenty of bulk to make you feel full. Fiber has another benefit. It helps to lower your cholesterol. Good sources of fiber are whole grains, fruits, vegetables, dried beans and legumes. Always drink 6 to 8 glasses of water per day when you are eating a high-fiber diet. For ways to increase the fiber content in your meals, see Chapter 4.

FIGURING IT OUT

How many calories per day should you eat to lose a certain amount of weight? Your dietitian can help you determine that number. The answer will depend on your present weight, your activity level, and the medications you take.

Following are two sample eating plans. The total calories in each are generally the daily amounts often recommended for adults trying to lose weight—1,200 calories for women, 1,500 calories for men. The first

1,200-CALORIE DAILY MENUS

HIGH-FAT, LOW-FIBER (LESS HEALTHFUL)	LOW-FAT, HIGH-FIBER (MORE HEALTHFUL)
Breakfast	
2 eggs	1 egg
2 slices bacon	1 slice Canadian bacon
2 pieces white toast with 1 tsp butter	2 pieces wheat toast, with low-sugar jelly and 1 tsp margarine
½ cup home fries	½ grapefruit
8 oz orange juice	
Lunch	
Hot dog on bun	2 oz sliced roast beef sandwich with lettuce, tomato, mustard
	Fresh peach
	3 cups plain popcorn
	½ cup coleslaw
Dinner	
McDonald's hamburger, regular size	McDonald's chicken sandwich
	2 orders of small salad with diet dressing
Nutrient Analysis	
Carbohydrate: 34%	Carbohydrate: 51% (goal: 50%–60%)
Protein: 17%	Protein: 21% (goal: 20%)
Fat: 49%	Fat: 28% (goal: 30%)

column shows a high-fat, low-fiber daily menu. The second column shows a menu with the same calorie count, but it has been modified to include more low-fat, high-fiber foods. Compare the two menus and you'll quickly see that the low-fat, high-fiber version is a much more balanced and filling meal plan—a model for healthy eating.

1,500-Calorie Daily Menus

HIGH-FAT, LOW-FIBER (LESS HEALTHFUL)	LOW-FAT, HIGH-FIBER (MORE HEALTHFUL)
Breakfast	
8 oz whole milk	8 oz low-fat (1%) milk
8 oz orange juice	½ banana
Doughnut	Whole-wheat English muffin with low-sugar jelly
	1 tbsp diet margarine
Lunch	
3 oz bologna sandwich with mayonnaise	2 oz turkey sandwich with lettuce, tomato, 1 tbsp diet mayonnaise
French fries, small serving	1 oz pretzels
	1 apple
Dinner	
½ cup broccoli with butter	½ cup broccoli with Butter Buds
4 oz hamburger patty	4 oz turkey patty
½ cup mashed potato	1 medium baked potato
	8-inch ear of corn
	Tossed salad with 2 tbsp diet salad dressing
Nutrient Analysis	
Carbohydrate: 32%	Carbohydrate: 50% (goal: 50%–60%)
Protein: 21%	Protein: 20% (goal: 20%)
Fat: 47%	Fat: 30% (goal: 30%)

Facts About Snacks

To help you manage your blood sugar levels, your dietitian may advise you to eat snacks between meals. The best snacks are those high in fiber and low in fat. Table 6-2 is a list of high-fiber, low-calorie snacks that can also keep you on the path to successful weight loss.

TABLE 6-2. HIGH-FIBER, LOW-CALORIE SNACKS

FOOD PRODUCT	FIBER	CALORIES
½ cup Fiber 1 cereal (or All-Bran with extra fiber) + ½ cup Dannon "light" yogurt	12 g	110
¾ cup raw raspberries + ½ cup low-fat cottage cheese	6.5 g	100
2 Wasa Fiber Plus crackers + ½ cup reduced-calorie American cheese	5.6 g	105
4 cups popcorn, air-popped (no added fat)	4 g	100
2 cups raw vegetables: combination of broccoli, carrots, celery + 2 tbsp low-calorie dressing	3.5 g	100
3 graham crackers	3 g	105
½ banana rolled in 2 tbsp Grapenuts cereal	3 g	115
3 Finn Crisp crackers + 1 tbsp "light" cream cheese	3 g	90
¾ cup blueberries + ½ cup Dannon "light" yogurt	3 g	110
½ cup cooked oat bran cereal + 1 tbsp raisins + cinnamon + artificial sweetener	4 g	110

Alcohol and Weight Loss

How do alcoholic beverages affect your weight-loss program? First of all, people with diabetes should never have more than one or two alcoholic drinks at a time, and only after getting their doctor's permission! That's because alcohol can affect your blood sugar levels, a topic discussed more fully in Chapter 21.

Right now, let's focus on alcohol's impact on your weight-loss program. Alcohol has calories that might slow your efforts. A 12-ounce light beer, an 8-ounce regular beer, 4 ounces of wine, or 1.5 ounces of "hard liquor" contain about 100 calories each. In addition, alcohol stimulates your appetite. If you're trying to lose weight, it's probably best to avoid alcohol entirely.

If you use insulin and occasionally want to have a drink, do not try to compensate for the calories in alcohol by cutting back on some other food in your meal plan. *If you do not use insulin*, by all means cut back on your calorie intake to account for a single cocktail on a special occasion. In either case, make sure you always eat some food when you drink alcohol to slow its passage into your bloodstream.

Healthy Food Tips

The following strategies can help you stick to a meal plan and lose weight:

- *Watch portion sizes.* The amount of any food you eat is very important to weight loss. For that reason, it's a good idea to weigh and measure your food. Keep a food scale, calculator, measuring cups and spoons in a handy spot in your kitchen. When eating away from home, remember that most restaurant portions are very large. Practice "eyeballing" your food at home to avoid overeating in a restaurant.
- *Put up reminders.* These notes can keep you true to your eating plan. Place them in a conspicuous spot—the door of the refrigerator or the bathroom mirror. Always write a positive message. Don't write: "Stay out of the refrigerator after work." Instead, write: "Snack on the carrot sticks in the crisper drawer." Notice the message is quite specific. It steers you directly to the proper snack without giving you the chance to think about other options.
- *Break chains of events that lead to overeating.* Lifestyle patterns that cause you to overeat often have nothing to do with food. For example, heavy traffic may lead to stress, causing you to stop at an ice cream parlor and overeat. This chain could be broken by taking an alternate route home to avoid heavy traffic and the ice cream parlor.
- *Break habits associated with overeating.* You may have developed behaviors that automatically lead to overeating. If watching TV prompts snacking, confine eating to areas away from the TV. If you

tend to eat very quickly—faster than the time your body needs to signal you are satisfied—put the utensils down between bites. Or pace your meal by serving salad as a first course.

- *Find activities to deal with the emotions that can lead to overeating.* Do you use food as a "comforter" when sad? As an "entertainer" when bored? As a "distracter" when under stress? Try to substitute some activity for eating at these times. Run errands when feeling restless, read a light fiction book when under stress, or telephone a friend when feeling lonely.
- *Ask for the support of family and friends.* If you tend to eat when preparing foods, perhaps others could cook for you. Or ask someone to encourage you with your weight-loss program. In sharing your goals with a friend, your commitment may rise dramatically.
- *Plan obstacles to unhealthy eating.* Make it hard to eat what you shouldn't. Place high-fat foods that others in the family may buy in places hard to reach—the back of a lower shelf of the refrigerator or the top of the kitchen cabinets, reachable only with a step-stool. Or put foods in containers you can't see through. Better yet, keep tempting sweets and high-fat foods out of your home entirely.
- *Plan aids to healthy eating.* Make it easy to eat what you should. Instead of "grazing" through the kitchen when you get home from work, have a lettuce salad or precut vegetables ready. Leave fresh fruit in plain sight, or carry an apple with you for the return trip. In essence, create your own low-fat environment.
- *Keep a food record.* Eat at every meal and snack time. Never skip a meal, a common weight-loss ploy that can have a negative effect on your blood sugar. If you don't eat a meal and your insulin is still active, your blood sugar may get too low. Each time you eat, record it in a notebook or diary, and at the end of the day, add up the total calories you have consumed that day. You'll get a psychological boost from seeing how well you are sticking to your meal plan that is helping you to both control your diabetes and lose weight.

EXERCISE—THE OTHER HALF OF THE EQUATION

Exercise is also an important part of managing diabetes. Exercise increases your body's sensitivity to insulin. And of course, if you are trying to lose weight, exercise can help you burn excess calories. But to develop healthy thinking about exercise, you should first squelch a few myths. For example, "no pain, no gain" implies that for exercise to be effective, you must endure pain. This simply isn't true. Your exercise program should make you feel good, not uncomfortable.

Another myth is that sporadic activity, such as running for a bus, is all the exercise you need. Again, this isn't true. Exercise periods should last at least 20 to 30 minutes, with sustained activity that boosts your heart rate and makes you breathe faster than normal—so-called aerobic exercise. Your body doesn't even start to burn fat until you reach the 20-minute mark, so to lose weight, a good rule of thumb for daily exercise is 40 to 45 minutes. Still other myths imply that exercise is only for young people who dance to music in fashionable leotards or jog in miserable weather. Not so! Your body, too, has muscles. Research has shown that everyone, old and young, can benefit immensely from aerobic exercise.

In beginning an exercise program to lose and then maintain your weight, always get clearance from your doctor first. Then talk with your exercise physiologist to develop a workable plan. Have a positive attitude about your exercise plan, pushing aside all negative thoughts. Exercise is not punishment for being overweight. It is not a necessary evil you must endure. Instead, it is a time you can claim just for yourself. Exercise helps you relax tense muscles and relieve stress. Best of all, it's a way of simply making you feel good.

Turn again to Chapter 5 to help plan your exercise program. And be sure to follow the safety tips on page 72. Then ease into your program, choosing activities you like. Be flexible and allow for occasional backsliding. A missed session shouldn't become an overblown issue that makes you throw in the towel. Some days are easier than others to carry out your plan. But if you make exercise a high priority, it will soon become a natural part of your day—as natural as eating and sleeping.

Here's a tip that will help you stay faithful to your program. When you are trying to lose weight, keep track of your progress by writing it down on a chart or in a notebook. When you achieve a certain goal, reward yourself. Go to a movie or buy yourself a present.

Burning Calories with Exercise

You can burn calories with exercise, the total amount depending on your weight and on how long and hard you exercise. Figure 6-1 will give you an idea of how many calories you can burn with 30 minutes of various types of exercise.

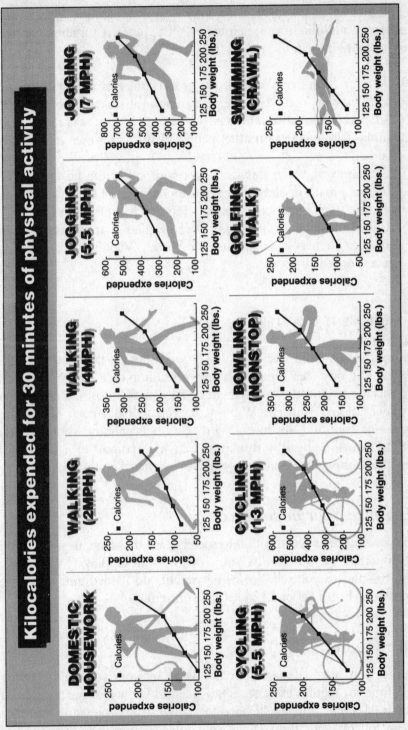

Kilocalories expended for 30 minutes of physical activity

Figure 6-1

You also can burn extra calories by simply adopting a more active lifestyle. In addition to your aerobic exercise, here are some ways to put more activity into your day:

- *Do errands on foot*. Walk to the grocery store or post office.
- *Walk the dog*. Your "best friend" can be a valuable exercise partner.
- *Rely less on mechanical devices*. Use a push lawnmower rather than riding. Also rely less on other people; deliver your own messages at work.
- *Use the worst parking spaces*. Park your car at the far end of the shopping mall, if safety allows; use the lot farthest from your office.
- *Use the stairs*. Stair-climbing is a top-notch calorie burner.
- *Redefine housework and yard work*. Rather than dreary chores, consider them a chance to burn off calories. Vacuuming and raking never looked so good!

COMMITMENT MATTERS

Knowing you should lose weight is a good start on the road to better health. The next step is commitment—deciding on a course of action and sticking to it until you reach your goal. But the most important step is understanding yourself. Without it, you will not even be able to begin—or continue—to lose weight. By understanding yourself, you can develop the "healthy thinking" that is important to a successful weight-loss program. Here are some key elements in that thinking:

Recognize Your Importance

Everyone makes a contribution to society, whether large or small. You are important to your family, your friends, your employer, your community—and to yourself. In losing weight, do it for those who care about you. But most of all, do it for yourself!

Take Control

Perhaps you have allowed your family to set your schedule, leaving little time for regular exercise. They need to know that for the sake of your well-being, things will have to change. Life's pressures can also take a toll on your time—work schedules, community activities, or other obligations. You should identify and take control of these pressures, rather than letting them control you.

Be Objective and Realistic

No one is asking you to run the marathon or lose 50 pounds in a week. Instead, set reasonable goals. Walk four blocks a day during the first week of your exercise program. Plan to lose ½ to 1 pound a week.

Stress the Positive

Look for positive ways to keep your commitment high. For example, *accept life's flaws.* Rather than abandoning your meal plan because you overate at one meal, learn from your failings and continue your program with confidence. *See things as they really are.* A single setback, such as twisting your ankle, should not doom your whole exercise program. Again, keep your eyes on your long-term goal. Rather than thinking that exercise takes too much of your time, see it as time you have for yourself that will make you look better, feel better, and get greater enjoyment out of your life.

Here is a checklist to help you stay true to your goals.

- *Consult your physician and health-care team.* They can help you set overall weight-loss goals and review how weight loss may affect your medication needs.

- *Establish an eating plan.* Your dietitian can help. And remember, this is your blueprint for a lifetime of healthy eating.

- *Set realistic goals.* Set goals you can control and meet. Write them down in a notebook. Include weekly exercise goals. Or goals for high-fiber foods to add to your diet and high-fat foods to resist. Avoid goals like "I will lose 2 pounds this week." You can't necessarily control that, given the many factors that influence weight from day to day. Instead, write something like "I will calculate the total calories I eat each day."

- *Keep a food diary and weight-loss chart.* A spiral notebook will do. Keep track of what you eat each day and plan a weekly weigh-in to record your weight. Plot your weight each week on a simple chart.

- *Establish an exercise plan.* First, see your physician for an OK. An exercise physiologist can help develop a workable routine that you can stick to.

- *Make sure you have blood glucose testing equipment and know how to use it.* Eating fewer calories and increasing exercise can lower your blood sugar. Make sure you test your blood sugar daily. Record the results along with your daily food diary. Be sure to contact your health-care team if your blood sugar levels are getting lower and a medication adjustment is needed.

- *Use measuring cups, spoons, and scales.* Watch those portions!

- *Get support.* Enlist the support of family and friends. It's great to have encouragement!

Research shows that despite some people's best efforts, they will never be successful at losing much weight. If you fall into this category, do not despair. You can still improve your blood sugar levels and decrease your risks for complications by exercising more, using your eating plan and medications consistently, and using home blood sugar monitoring to keep track of your results and make adjustments as needed.

Part Three

TREATING DIABETES WITH MEDICATIONS

CHAPTER 7

Diabetes Pills

SOME PEOPLE WITH DIABETES need medications to bring their blood sugar into good control. Others do not; they can keep their diabetes in control with nutrition and exercise. Depending on your body's needs, your doctor may prescribe medications to help you manage your blood sugar. Among them are *oral hypoglycemic medications*, often called "diabetes pills," which are used in combination with meal planning and exercise programs to lower your blood sugar. Diabetes pills are prescribed for certain people with Type II diabetes. If you have Type I diabetes, these pills will not be a part of your treatment.

WHAT ARE DIABETES PILLS?

Diabetes pills are medications for diabetes that are taken orally—by mouth. These pills *do not contain insulin*. Currently, insulin exists only in a liquid form that must be injected. In other words, diabetes pills are not a tablet form of insulin. Instead, they are medications that help the body make or release its *own* insulin and help the body use insulin more effectively.

Who Can Take Diabetes Pills?

Diabetes pills aren't for everyone with diabetes. They're effective only if your pancreas is still capable of producing insulin; your body just needs a "boost" to increase its ability to produce insulin and to use it more effectively. This means that some people—those with Type I diabetes and those with Type II diabetes whose bodies have lost the ability to produce sufficient insulin—cannot use diabetes pills. Pills are most likely to be effective in people who developed Type II diabetes after age 40 and who have had it for less than 10 years.

How Do Diabetes Pills Work?

Diabetes pills work by stimulating the pancreas, the organ that makes insulin. They also work actively in the liver and other cells of the body.

- They help your pancreas release more insulin.
- They help decrease your cells' resistance to insulin. This means that even though the amount of insulin produced by your body may be lower than normal, it may still be enough to handle your blood sugar.
- They increase the sensitivity of the insulin receptors on the cells, allowing your body to get by with lower amounts of insulin.
- They prevent the release of too much stored glucose from the liver, which would overload the bloodstream with more glucose than the available insulin could handle.

It's important to note that there are wide differences in people with Type II diabetes. In many people with this type of diabetes, the pancreas does not produce enough insulin. But some people with Type II diabetes actually produce *more* insulin than normal; their body just can't use it effectively. Overall, however, these medications enable some people with diabetes to use their own insulin more effectively throughout the entire day. This is particularly true for people who follow a meal plan and exercise regularly.

How to Take Diabetes Pills

If you use diabetes pills, there are two basic rules you should follow:

- Diabetes pills should be taken before or with meals.
- Skipped doses should not be made up. If you accidentally miss a dose, simply wait to take a pill at the next appropriate time.

TYPES OF DIABETES PILLS

SULFONYLUREAS. In the United States, there are two major classes of diabetes pills—*sulfonylureas* and *biguanides*. Within the sulfonylurea class, there are two main types:

1. Those that have been available for many years, known as "first generation."
2. A more recent group, known as "second-generation" medications.

Table 7-1 lists the various types of sulfonylureas available in the United States. If you need to take diabetes pills, your physician will prescribe the best type for your particular situation.

Sulfonylureas are commonly prescribed to be taken before meals. The exact meals and time before the meals vary from pill to pill. Occasionally, sulfonylureas may be given along with insulin or other diabetes medications. Combining two types of sulfonylurea pills does not usually increase their effectiveness, however. If you use a sulfonylurea and forget to take your pills, do not take the additional pills later in the day. Unless advised otherwise, it is usually safer to have your blood sugar run a little high temporarily than to risk a low-sugar reaction.

BIGUANIDES. Biguanides are the other class of oral agents used in the United States, and in fact have just recently come into use here. These drugs may be helpful for people who have been using sulfonylureas for a period of time and who find they are becoming less effective in controlling blood sugars. They have been used in Europe and other parts of the world for a while. *Metformin* is the only oral medication available in this class of drugs. Metformin may be used alone or in combination with a sulfonylurea or insulin. Table 7-1 provides some additional information on metformin. Always check with your physician and health-care team about combining any medications.

Table 7-1. Oral Hypoglycemic Medications in Use in the United States

Generic Name	Trade Name	Manufacturer	Tablet	Usual Daily Dose
"First-Generation" Sulfonylurea Agents				
Tolbutamide	Orinase	generic	White 500 mg	500–2000 mg
Tolazamide	Tolinase	generic	White 100 mg / White 250 mg / White 500 mg	100–1000 mg
Chlorpropamide	Diabinese	Pfizer	Blue 100 mg / Blue 250 mg	100–500 mg (occ. 750 mg)
"Second-Generation" Sulfonylurea Agents				
Glipizide	Glucotrol	Roerig Div. of Pfizer	White 5 mg / White 10 mg	2.5–40 mg
Glipizide GITS	Glucotrol XL	Pfizer	White 5 mg / White 10 mg	5–20 mg

Drug	Brand	Manufacturer	Color/Strength	Dose Range
Glyburide (glybenclamide)	Micronase	Upjohn	White 1.25 mg / Pink 2.5 mg / Blue 5 mg	1.25–20 mg
	Glynase Press Tabs	Upjohn	White 1.5 mg / Blue 3 mg	1.5–12 mg
	Diabeta	Hoechst-Roussel	White 1.25 mg / Pink 2.5 mg / Light Green 5 mg	1.25–20 mg
Biguanides				
Metformin	Glucophage	Lipha/Bristol-Myers-Squibb	White 500 mg / White 850 mg	500–2500 mg / 850–2550 mg

Adapted and updated from the *Joslin Diabetes Manual*, Richard S. Beaser, M.D., and Leo Krall, M.D., Lea & Febiger, Philadelphia, 1989.

POSSIBLE SIDE EFFECTS

Although oral medications can be very effective in the treatment of diabetes, you need to be aware of some possible side effects.

Low Blood Sugar

First of all, your oral medication may do its job "too well," stimulating your pancreas to produce more insulin than is actually needed. As the excess insulin reacts with available sugar in the bloodstream, your blood sugar may dip abnormally low (below 60 mg/dl), resulting in low blood sugar or *hypoglycemia*. This is more likely to occur with a sulfonylurea than with metformin.

Any medication that lowers your blood sugar must be used carefully to ensure that the level does not dip too low. For example, exercise lowers blood sugar. You therefore need to time your diabetes pills, exercise, and meals appropriately, so that there is enough food and not too much medication to cause such a dip in your blood sugar.

However, low blood sugar may develop even when you do follow your program carefully—perhaps even *because* you are careful in your eating and exercise programs. Weight loss, for instance, may reduce your cells' resistance to insulin, causing you to need less insulin. Therefore, if you take diabetes pills and lose weight, be alert to the fact that your medication may have to be reduced or discontinued altogether.

Early signs of low blood sugar include hunger, shakiness, nervousness, sweating, dizziness, weakness, irritability, and heart pounding. If these symptoms develop, test your blood sugar, and if it's low follow the steps for responding to low blood sugar in Chapter 12. If the symptoms don't subside within 30 minutes, contact a member of your health-care team who can advise you about the proper dose and timing of your diabetes pills. The solution may involve taking a shorter-acting or longer-acting form of medication, depending on your eating and activity schedule.

Other Side Effects

Diabetes pills can occasionally cause other side effects. These include stomach and intestinal upsets, loss of appetite, skin rashes, and itching. If you experience these or other unusual side effects, notify your physician. Sometimes facial flushing occurs due to the combined effect of alcohol and a diabetes pill called *chlorpropamide* (Diabinese). This reaction can be frightening, but it is quite harmless. If you take this drug and have this reaction, your doctor may want to switch you to one of the newer second-generation drugs, which are less likely to cause problems when combined with alcohol or other drugs.

Many side effects will disappear as your body "adjusts" to your medications, but occasionally the dose needs to be reduced. In a few cases, people cannot tolerate a certain kind of medication, and a different type of pill should be prescribed. You should also watch for undesired side effects that may develop from combining diabetes pills with any other medications you may be taking. Other medications may cause your diabetes pills to lose some of their effectiveness. Medications that can have this undesired result include certain diuretics, corticosteroids, birth control pills, and estrogen supplements. The best way to avoid any of these problems is to be sure your physician knows *all* the medications you are taking.

WHY DIABETES PILLS CAN FAIL

When used properly, diabetes pills can be very effective. For some people with Type II diabetes, however, the pills never work at all, not even in the beginning of their treatment. This is called "primary failure," and it is not clear why it happens, but in some people it may simply be that they did not have Type II diabetes, as suspected. They may have Type I diabetes that developed at an older age and as a result their bodies are making hardly any insulin or no insulin at all.

For unknown reasons, diabetes pills work for a while in some people but then lose their effectiveness. This is called "secondary failure," and it occurs gradually at the rate of 5 to 10 percent per year, perhaps because the body is producing less insulin or becoming more resistant to its own naturally produced insulin. Sometimes secondary failure is triggered by an infection, disease, or emotional stress. In such cases, the person may require insulin injections until the problem is resolved and eventually may return to using just the diabetes pills. When one type of pill becomes ineffective, the doctor may switch to another drug. With the recent addition of metformin to the list of drug choices, a pill that works differently from the sulfonylureas is available for you to try if your existing medications begin to work less well.

Sometimes the failure of diabetes pills is due not to the medications themselves, but because of "user error." People often make the mistake of abandoning their meal plan or exercise program, believing the tablets alone will handle their diabetes. But as effective as these pills may be, they can't take care of your diabetes by themselves. For this reason, a disciplined program—one that includes a meal plan and regular exercise—is extremely important. In fact, the difference between success and failure will depend on whether a sensible program is followed.

If you take oral medications for your diabetes, work with your health-care team to develop a meal plan and exercise program. Then resolve to do your best to follow them. In the long run, attention to *all aspects* of your treatment program can help improve your diabetes control. Some people find that they eventually can stop taking their diabetes pills altogether, relying solely on nutrition and exercise to keep their blood sugar in control.

OTHER MEDICATIONS

Many people with diabetes cannot take oral medications. They need to take insulin, which is available only in liquid form and must be injected. However, scientists are trying to overcome this obstacle. Researchers are also working to develop other pills to lower blood sugars. Several promising drugs are now being studied that boost insulin production, help insulin work better, or help reduce the amount of sugar that is absorbed in your bloodstream. Ask your health-care team to keep you informed about these advances. Continue to learn all you can about diabetes. The more you know, the better you will be at working to achieve a truly effective treatment program.

CHAPTER 8

Insulin Therapy

SCIENTISTS TEND TO USE the word *breakthrough* very sparingly, saving it for the most remarkable advances. But certainly the discovery of insulin can be categorized as a breakthrough—one of the greatest medical achievements of all time. During the past century, this medication has improved and saved the lives of millions of people who cannot produce enough insulin to meet their body's needs. If you are among that group, your doctor may prescribe insulin to help you restore and maintain more normal blood glucose levels. Used in conjunction with nutrition and exercise, insulin can improve the quality of your life immeasurably.

THE STORY OF INSULIN

Insulin treatment has been available for less than 75 years. Before then, many people died from diabetes; or if they had Type II diabetes, they lived for a number of years but functioned very poorly. But thanks to the efforts of two Canadian doctors, Frederick Banting and Charles Best, insulin was first extracted from the pancreases of animals in 1921 and injected into animals that had diabetes. The experiments were a dramatic success. Within a year, insulin was being used to treat humans.

Over the years, there have been several changes in the way insulin is manufactured. Until recently, the insulins produced in the United States were made from animal insulin. They were extracted from the pancreases of cattle or pigs, or were a mixture of the two. For most users, this animal-based insulin was quite acceptable. But some people experienced side effects from these early insulins, due to impurities and the fact that the insulin was from animals. For example, some developed allergic responses, which could vary from a slight redness and itching to considerable swelling and pain at the injection site. In fact, the immune system of some individuals actually perceived the insulin as a foreign substance, and their bodies responded by making antibodies to counteract the injected insulin. People who had this reaction sometimes developed resistance to the action of insulin and then required unusually large doses.

Fortunately, manufacturers have developed ways to remove most of the impurities from animal insulin. Today, highly purified animal insulins are available, and side effects have been significantly reduced.

Recently, scientists revolutionized the production of insulin even further by developing synthetic *human* insulin. It is identical with the insulin produced by the human body; because it is not produced by animals but through "genetic engineering," its structure is identical with what a person's own pancreas would make if it could. Today, most of the insulin used in the United States is of this type.

FACTS ABOUT INSULIN

To manage your diabetes effectively, you need to know some basic facts about insulin:

- Insulin must be injected. It cannot be taken orally (by mouth) because insulin is digested by the stomach juices, which destroy its effectiveness.
- Insulin is measured in "units," often designated by the letter U.
- Insulin is produced in two different *strengths* in the United States— U-100 and U-500. The vast majority of people use U-100, which means there are 100 units of insulin in each cubic centimeter (cc) of liquid (a cubic centimeter is about the size of a small sugar cube). You must use the proper syringe to measure the correct dose. For example, a U-100 syringe must be used to measure units of U-100 insulin. (People living in or traveling to other countries may find other strengths as well.)
- In addition to different *strengths* of insulin, there are three different *types* of insulin—short-acting, intermediate-acting, and long-acting. These types of insulin vary in three important ways, all relating to *time:* (1) how quickly the insulin starts to work (onset);

(2) when the insulin works the hardest (peak activity); and (3) how long the insulin continues to work (duration).

TYPES OF INSULIN

When insulin was first made available, people with diabetes had no choice of the type they could use. Only one type was available. It was short-acting, working over a brief period of time without much variation. The standard treatment was to take several injections a day. Later, another type became available. This was a longer-acting insulin, which made it possible to decrease the number of daily injections. Today, there are three different types of insulin, all varying in the *timing* of their work and how they are used in treatment.

To appreciate this, think about how the body normally works. Before you had diabetes, your blood sugar levels were maintained within the normal range by a slow continuous secretion of natural insulin from the pancreas into the blood (the "basal" insulin supply). This kept the glucose level within the normal range (60–140 mg/dl or 60–110 mg/dl before a meal). And when you needed extra insulin, such as at meals, the pancreas provided additional bursts. Thus, insulin levels in your blood were changed automatically as needed.

Now that you have diabetes, the match between injected insulin and your body's needs is not as finely tuned as it was when your pancreas was working normally. With injected insulin, a certain amount of time must pass before it begins working. It then reaches a peak of effectiveness, after which it tapers off. Thus, your insulin needs may not always coincide with this pattern of insulin activity.

The difficulty of matching injected insulin with your body's needs is caused by many factors. The rate that insulin is absorbed may be affected by factors such as

- the type of insulin
- the injection site (such as the arm or leg)
- the depth of the injection
- and even the temperature of the skin and surrounding air

Variations in your meals—including the time you eat, and the amount and type of food consumed—also can contribute to a mismatch.

Despite these difficulties, you should make every effort to keep your blood glucose levels as close to normal as possible, throughout the day and night. The different types of insulin—short-acting, intermediate-acting, and long-acting—can help you in this effort. You and your health-care team can develop a daily insulin plan that fits your meal plan and exercise program. Please note that the times listed in the following discussion of each one of these insulins are *ranges*. Timing actually varies from person to person, and it tends to be on the shorter part of the range with human insulin than with animal-source insulins.

Short-Acting Insulin

Short-acting insulin begins working within 30–60 minutes of injection. It works hardest 2–4 hours after injection (the "peak" time) and is completely gone after 6–8 hours. If you are totally dependent on insulin and use only short-acting insulin, you would need an injection every 6 hours. The pattern of short-acting insulin is shown in Figure 8-1.

The most common form of short-acting insulin is called "regular" and comes in a clear solution.

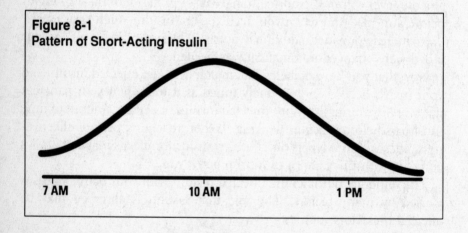

Figure 8-1
Pattern of Short-Acting Insulin

7 AM   10 AM   1 PM

Intermediate-Acting Insulin

Intermediate-acting insulins begin to work within 1–3 hours of injection. They reach their peak in 6–12 hours and may continue to work for up to 18–26 hours after injection. Their action pattern is shown in Figure 8-2.

One form of intermediate-acting insulin is called NPH, which stands for "Neutral Protamine Hagedorn." Protamine is a protein added to regular insulin which delays insulin's absorption from under the skin,

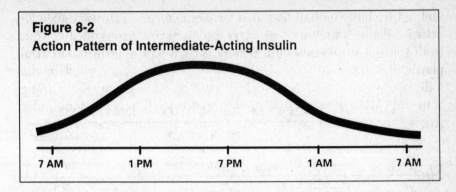

Figure 8-2
Action Pattern of Intermediate-Acting Insulin

7 AM   1 PM   7 PM   1 AM   7 AM

making it work over a longer period of time. Hagedorn is the name of the person who developed this type of insulin.

Another form of intermediate-acting insulin is called "Lente" (slow). It is made by adding zinc to regular insulin, which forms crystals which slow the rate of its absorption into the bloodstream, prolonging its action. Both NPH and Lente have a cloudy appearance.

Long-Acting Insulin

Long-acting insulin doesn't begin working until 4–8 hours after injection. It has a relatively low, prolonged peak, which occurs 12–18 hours after injection, and continues to work for up to 24–28 hours. There is one form of long-acting insulin, Ultralente, which is also made by adding zinc to prolong its activity, producing a cloudy solution. Figure 8-3 shows the action pattern of long-acting insulin.

Long-acting insulin is used in combination with an injection of regular insulin before each meal. This usually means you would have to have three shots a day (one mixed dose of regular/Ultralente at breakfast; regular insulin at lunch, and a mixed dose of regular/Ultralente at din-

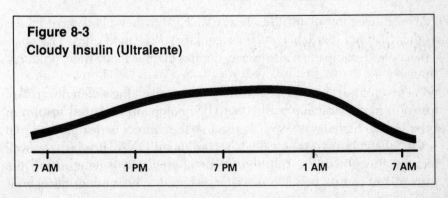

Figure 8-3
Cloudy Insulin (Ultralente)

7 AM   1 PM   7 PM   1 AM   7 AM

ner). Ultralente is often used in a form of diabetes treatment called "intensive diabetes therapy," which is discussed in Chapter 9.

Table 8-1 summarizes the activity of each type of insulin—its onset, peak, and duration.

TABLE 8-1. SUMMARY OF THE ACTIVITY OF INSULIN TYPES

	SHORT-ACTING (REGULAR)	INTERMEDIATE-ACTING (NPH, LENTE)	LONG-ACTING (ULTRALENTE, HUMAN)
Onset	approximately ½ hour	1–3 hours	approx. 4–8 hours
Peak	2–4 hours	6–12 hours	approx. 12–18 hours
Duration	6–8 hours	18–26 hours	approx. 24–28 hours

Mixed Doses of Insulins

As the peak activities of short-acting, intermediate-acting, and long-acting insulins are different, they can often be combined in a single injection called a *mixed dose*. Mixed insulin doses give your body an early peak to cover the meal eaten right after the injection and also provide prolonged insulin activity to take you through the day or night.

Commonly, short-acting (regular) insulin is mixed with intermediate-acting or long-acting insulin. Intermediate-acting is rarely mixed with long-acting insulin. When regular and intermediate insulins are taken at the same time, the intermediate-acting insulin begins to work the hardest just as the short-acting insulin subsides. The activity pattern of these two insulins working together is shown in Figure 8-4.

Brands of Insulin

A wide selection of insulins is available, and they often have names other than familiar labels such as regular, NPH, and Lente. The pharmaceutical companies also make varying claims about their products' purity.

The chart at the end of the chapter describes the different types of insulin made available by the two U.S. companies that sell insulin in the United States as of 1995. It also lists the sources of insulin—animal or synthetic human (also called "recombinant DNA" insulin)—as well as the strength of the solution. Your physician will recommend the brand you should use. Do not change brands without consulting your

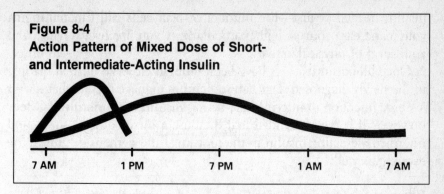

Figure 8-4
**Action Pattern of Mixed Dose of Short-
and Intermediate-Acting Insulin**

7 AM   1 PM   7 PM   1 AM   7 AM

doctor. Even minor differences in the makeup of the insulin may alter
the effectiveness of your treatment program.

CHOICE AND DOSE OF INSULIN

Initially, it may be impossible for your health-care team to predict the
exact dose of insulin you need. To some extent, the dose is determined
by trial and error. But once an appropriate dose is established, unless
instructed otherwise, you should use the *same amount* at the *same time*
each day. In deciding how to prescribe your insulin, your health-care
team will consider many factors, including the type of diabetes you
have. Each type requires a different approach.

Type I Diabetes

Type I diabetes (insulin-dependent) usually develops in four main
stages—*newly diagnosed, remission, intensification,* and *total diabetes.*
Each of these stages can have an impact on the type and timing of your
insulin doses.

NEWLY DIAGNOSED. During this stage, you still have some beta cells
that can produce insulin, but not enough to meet all your insulin
needs. But remember, your body has not had enough insulin during
the days or weeks prior to your diagnosis. To restore your body to
normal functioning after this period without enough insulin, your doctor may initially prescribe large doses of insulin. For example, high
levels of sugar and ketones in your blood may have reduced the ability
of your cells to respond to insulin. This means your initial doses may
have to be higher. Other factors can also influence the amount of

insulin needed at first—the number of beta cells still functioning in your pancreas, your weight (particularly if you are overweight), and your level of physical activity.

Once blood sugar levels have been brought closer to normal, people in the newly diagnosed stage can sometimes manage their diabetes with a single injection of intermediate-acting insulin each morning. Often, however, it is recommended that they use a mixed dose of short- and intermediate-acting insulin in the morning, and perhaps insulin in the evening as well.

REMISSION. Once your blood glucose is lowered, the response of your body and its remaining beta cells usually improves. This may result in a period called *remission*, a "honeymoon" stage during which your diabetes subsides. People in this stage often manage their diabetes with small amounts of insulin each day. In this stage, you should continue your injections—even if your insulin needs are very small. If you stop and later restart when your diabetes intensifies, you may have an allergic response to insulin. Continuation of insulin treatment during this phase helps to prolong the beta cells' ability to make insulin.

INTENSIFICATION. During the third stage, called *intensification*, the few remaining beta cells in your pancreas are being destroyed by your immune system and are steadily losing their ability to produce insulin, causing a gradual increase in your blood sugar levels. During this stage, your doctor will have to progressively increase your insulin dose. The type and amount will depend on your individual needs. Perhaps you will have to take a greater number of daily injections as well.

TOTAL DIABETES. Once the stage of *total diabetes* is reached, the beta cells have been completely destroyed. At that time, most people with Type I diabetes will require at least two to three injections a day, often a mixture of short- and intermediate-acting insulin, or a combination of short-acting (regular) and long-acting (Ultralente). An example of one such program has as the first injection a mixture of short-acting and intermediate-acting insulin, given at least 30 minutes before breakfast. This allows the short-acting insulin to begin working at about the same time that the nutrients from your food enter your bloodstream, and prevents your blood sugar from rising too high after eating breakfast. The second injection of regular insulin is given 30 minutes before the evening meal. The third injection, usually intermediate-acting insulin, is given at bedtime. While this program is commonly used and effective for many people, there are other common injection schedules that your physician may recommend for you.

Type II Diabetes

Many people with Type II diabetes can manage their condition with meal planning, exercise, and in some cases, diabetes pills that stimulate the pancreas to produce more insulin. Such approaches often work for some time. Eventually, however, this strategy may not be sufficient. A combination of factors may worsen your diabetes. These include beta cells that are defective or reduced in numbers, or an increasing tendency of your body's cells to resist the effects of insulin. When these changes occur, you may need daily injections of insulin.

The amount of insulin needed by people with Type II diabetes varies from person to person. It also may change over time. Some people can manage their condition with a dose of intermediate-acting insulin before breakfast. Others may need a mixed dose of short- and intermediate-acting insulin before breakfast. Some people have to add a dose of intermediate-acting insulin at bedtime, and others need a mixed dose of short- and intermediate-acting insulin before breakfast and dinner. Some may use a schedule similar to the one described earlier for people with Type I diabetes. Still others may take intermediate-acting insulin at bedtime and diabetes pills in the morning.

MEASURING AND INJECTING INSULIN

To take insulin, you should learn how to measure and inject a proper dose. Insulin is injected by syringe into the fatty tissue beneath the skin. Recommended injection sites include the abdomen, upper buttocks, the back of the arms, and the front of the legs. These sites are shown in Figure 8-5.

Because different sites on your body vary in their absorption of insulin, the choice of sites may affect your blood sugar control. To decrease fluctuations in your blood sugar, it's best to have a "site-rotation" plan. One option is to rotate sites in one area such as the abdomen. Another plan takes into consideration the fact that insulin is absorbed more quickly in the abdomen than in the arms, and even more slowly in the thighs and hips. With this in mind, a person could inject in the

Figure 8-5
Injection Sites

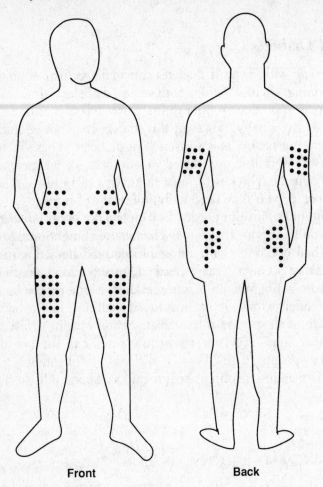

Front   Back

abdomen or arms in the morning (when blood sugars are usually highest), and inject in the thigh or upper area of the buttocks in the evening (when insulin is needed to last longer overnight).

To promote optimal insulin absorption, a general rule of thumb is to always rotate the injection site. This will reduce risk of *hypertrophy*, a mound of fat and fibrous tissue that develops from repeated injections in the same area.

There are two methods for measuring insulin for injection. The method you use depends on whether you are taking one or two types of insulin. A dose using one type of insulin is a "single dose." A dose using two types is called a "mixed dose" and involves short-acting insulin (clear) and intermediate-acting (cloudy) insulin. Instructions for administering a single dose are illustrated below.

How to administer a single dose:

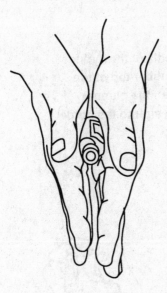

Figure 8-6a
Roll the insulin bottle between the palms of your hands, upside down, and sideways. Wipe off the bottle top with a cotton swab soaked with rubbing alcohol, or a pre-packaged alcohol wipe.

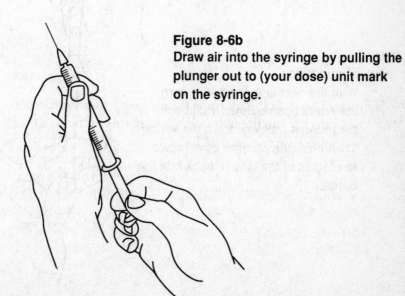

Figure 8-6b
Draw air into the syringe by pulling the plunger out to (your dose) unit mark on the syringe.

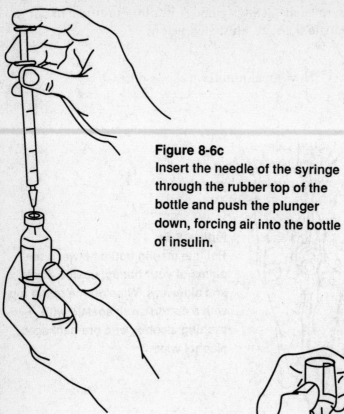

Figure 8-6c
Insert the needle of the syringe
through the rubber top of the
bottle and push the plunger
down, forcing air into the bottle
of insulin.

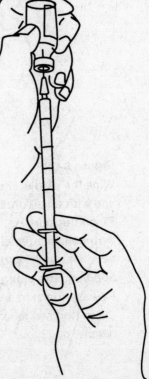

Figure 8-6d
With the needle in the bottle, turn
the bottle upside down. Pull back
the plunger halfway down the syringe.
Then push the plunger down again,
forcing all of the insulin back into the
bottle.

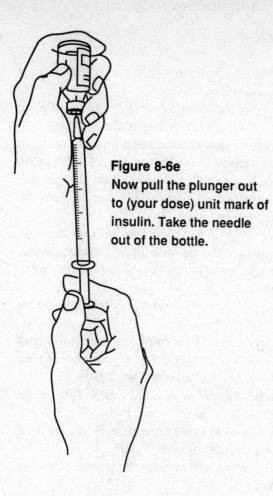

Figure 8-6e
Now pull the plunger out to (your dose) unit mark of insulin. Take the needle out of the bottle.

Figure 8-6f
Wipe the skin of the injection site with an alcohol swab. Pinch the skin. Holding the syringe like a pencil, push the needle straight into the skin and push the plunger down. Release the skin and, pressing the cotton swab next to the needle, pull it out.

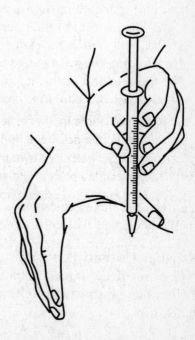

Instructions for Mixed Dose

1. Roll the "cloudy" bottle of insulin between the palms of your hands, upside down, and sideways.
2. Wipe off the tops of both the "cloudy" and "clear" bottles of insulin with an alcohol swab or prepackaged alcohol wipe.
3. Pull the plunger out to (*your dose of cloudy insulin*) unit mark on the syringe. Insert the needle through the top of the cloudy bottle, keeping the bottle upright on a table. Push the plunger down, forcing air into the bottle. Remove the needle from the bottle (the syringe and needle are empty).
4. Pull the plunger out to (*your dose of clear insulin*) unit mark on the syringe. Insert the needle through the top of the clear bottle, keeping the bottle upright on a table. Push the plunger down, forcing air into the bottle.
5. Leave the needle in the clear bottle and turn the bottle upside down.
6. Pull the plunger halfway down. Then push all the insulin back into the bottle. Now pull the plunger back to (*your dose of clear insulin*) unit mark of insulin and take out the needle.
7. Turn the cloudy bottle upside down and insert the needle through the rubber top.
8. Pull the plunger slowly back to (*your clear dose + cloudy dose*) unit mark. Remove the needle from the bottle.
9. Wipe the skin of the injection site with a cotton swab soaked in alcohol. Pinch the skin.
10. Holding the syringe like a pencil, push the needle straight into the skin and push the plunger down.
11. Release the skin and, pressing the cotton swab next to the needle, pull it out.

CARE AND STORAGE OF EQUIPMENT

You can purchase disposable plastic syringes in most pharmacies. In many states, you will need a prescription from your physician.

STORING UNUSED BOTTLES. Labels on insulin bottles say: *Store in cold place.* Keep unused bottles in your refrigerator. Avoid freezing. Follow these instructions for unopened bottles, not those you are currently using.

STORING BOTTLES CURRENTLY IN USE. Most people find it uncomfortable to inject cold insulin. Bottles you are currently using may be stored at room temperature. Temperature extremes should be avoided. Keep the insulin out of direct sunlight and away from radiators or other warm locations. Do not store insulin near ice or allow it to freeze.

EXPIRATION DATE. Insulin bottles are marked with an expiration date. Once that date has passed, the manufacturer will not guarantee its effectiveness. Regardless of the expiration date, insulin stored at room temperature begins to lose some of its potency after a month and should be discarded, even if some insulin remains.

EXTRA BOTTLES. You should keep at least one extra bottle of each type of insulin you use on hand at all times. Extra bottles should be stored in the refrigerator to retain potency. The butter or egg compartment is a convenient storage place.

CARING FOR SYRINGES. Disposable syringes are designed to be used once and then discarded. To save money, however, some people use a syringe two or three times. In such cases, you should recap the syringe. Then store it in a dry spot, and if you are reusing, do so within 24 hours.

DISPOSING OF SYRINGES. Get rid of your syringes by placing them in a coffee can or some other container that can be closed tightly and stored in a safe place. This is especially important if you have children in your home. When the container is full, add bleach, tape closed, and dispose of according to local regulations. Never discard "loose" syringes. Someone might get stuck accidentally, leading to infection.

TRAVELING WITH INSULIN. When traveling, keep your insulin and syringes with you. This will prevent the possibility of your supplies being misplaced. More suggestions for caring for your diabetes while traveling will be discussed in Chapter 22.

ALTERNATIVE INJECTION DEVICES. Some people use other types of devices to inject insulin. For example, a small *automatic injector* may be used. With this device, the syringe is filled with insulin as usual and placed in the injector, and then the injector is spring-cocked. After the injection site has been cleaned, the injector is set against the skin. The person touches a small trigger, and the device forces the needle through the skin. The person then pushes the plunger down, injecting insulin.

Button infusers are made up of little injectable discs attached to a catheter, or tubing, that leads to a needle inserted beneath the skin. *Jet injectors* are also available. These use no needles, but force insulin through the skin using air under great pressure. Some people use *insulin pumps*, devices that will be discussed in more detail in Chapter 9. For people with poor eyesight, there are syringe magnifiers, insulin gauges, and "click-count" syringes and syringe "pens" that count out unit measurements of insulin to improve the accuracy of doses.

Medical Frontiers

While insulin has been a "wonder drug" for many years, no one enjoys getting injections day after day. That's why scientists are working to develop a form of insulin that can be taken by mouth which would be easier to use and possibly less expensive, too. They are also studying a nose spray that contains insulin. In addition, they are trying to develop new forms of insulin that act over different time periods and may be even more effective than human insulin.

Other research is focusing on beta-cell transplants in which normal beta cells from a carefully matched donor are given to a diabetes patient to revitalize the recipient's pancreas. Pancreas transplants are being studied. And devices that are implanted into the body are also being investigated. Other scientists are trying to pinpoint the genes that contribute to diabetes. They eventually hope to find ways to correct these genetic flaws, working to prevent diabetes in people at high risk for the disease.

One of the most significant advances in recent years was a 10-year study completed in 1993, called the Diabetes Control and Complications Trial (DCCT). This study answered the question that has been asked almost since the discovery of insulin: When is diabetes control *good enough* to actually slow or prevent long-term complications? How good is good? The study has shown that if people with diabetes keep their blood sugar as close as possible to the levels enjoyed by people who do not have diabetes, they will develop fewer chronic complications. In other words, people who take the time to monitor their blood sugar levels 4 to 5 times a day and make adjustments in their medication, exercise, and nutrition—keeping their blood sugar levels as normal as possible—will decrease the risk of problems with their eyes, nerves, and kidneys by 50 percent or more. This exciting news points to the benefits of a treatment called *intensive diabetes therapy*, the subject of Chapter 9.

AVAILABLE INSULINS

PRODUCT	MANUFACTURER	SOURCE	STRENGTH
Short-acting Insulins			
Humulin Regular	Lilly	Human	U-100
Novolin R (Regular)	Novo	Human	U-100
Novolin R Penfill (Regular)	Novo	Human	U-100
Velosulin Human (Regular)	Novo	Human	U-100
Iletin II Regular	Lilly	Pork	U-100, U-500
Purified Pork R (Regular)	Novo	Pork	U-100
Velosulin (Regular)	Novo	Pork	U-100
Iletin I Regular	Lilly	Beef/Pork	U-40, U-100
Regular	Novo	Pork	U-100
Intermediate-acting Insulins			
Humulin L (Lente)	Lilly	Human	U-100
Humulin N (NPH)	Lilly	Human	U-100
Insulatard Human (NPH)	Novo	Human	U-100
Novolin L (Lente)	Novo	Human	U-100
Novolin N (NPH)	Novo	Human	U-100
Novolin N Penfill (NPH)	Novo	Human	U-100
Iletin II Lente	Lilly	Pork	U-100
Iletin II NPH	Lilly	Pork	U-100
Insulatard NPH	Novo	Pork	U-100
Purified Pork Lente	Novo	Pork	U-100
Purified Pork N (NPH)	Novo	Pork	U-100
Lente	Novo	Beef	U-100
Iletin I Lente	Lilly	Beef/Pork	U-40, U-100
Iletin I NPH	Lilly	Beef/Pork	U-40, U-100
NPH	Novo	Beef	U-100

AVAILABLE INSULINS (continued)

PRODUCT	MANUFACTURER	SOURCE	STRENGTH
Long-acting Insulins			
Humulin U (Ultralente)	Lilly	Human	U-100
Ultralente	Novo	Beef/Pork	U-100
*Mixtures**			
Mixtard (30% Regular, 70% NPH)	Novo	Pork	U-100
Mixtard (70% NPH, 30% Regular)	Novo	Human	U-100
Novolin 70/30 (70% NPH, 30% Regular)	Novo	Human	U-100
Novolin 70/30 Penfill (70% NPH, 30% Regular)	Novo	Human	U-100
Humulin 70/30 (70% NPH, 30% Regular)	Lilly	Human	U-100
Humulin 50/50	Lilly	Human	U-100

* More mixtures may be available.

CHAPTER 9

Intensive Diabetes Therapy

THE INSULIN THERAPY DISCUSSED in the previous chapter is often called *"conventional"* *diabetes therapy*. This form of treatment is the standard, or usual, approach to treating diabetes with insulin. It usually involves one to three insulin injections each day, testing your blood sugar, and following a meal plan. The doses of insulin are generally "fixed," that is, unchanged from day to day.

There's also a form of treatment called *"intensive"* *diabetes therapy*, or *intensive insulin therapy*. In this approach, the idea is to mimic the way a normal pancreas would respond to the body's need for insulin. It involves frequent testing of your blood sugar and adjustment to your insulin dose or meal plan. In fact, the insulin doses or meal plan may change from one day to the next.

Intensive diabetes therapy is being used more and more these days, due to the availability of self-testing devices that accurately measure blood sugar levels. This form of therapy is not for everyone. Many people who use insulin manage quite well with conventional therapy. Nonetheless, you may be a good candidate for intensive therapy. The previously mentioned Diabetes Control and Complications Trial has now concluded that intensive therapy is better than conventional therapy in preventing long-term complications of diabetes. It does, however, increase the risk of having low blood sugar.

A MATTER OF DEGREE

For decades, conventional insulin therapy has been the cornerstone of care for millions of people who need insulin. It is a proven way to manage your blood sugar. In fact, intensive insulin therapy is not really a different form of treatment for diabetes at all. Rather, it is another way of using the conventional treatment. As a result, there may not be a clear dividing line between the two types, only a difference of degree. Also a difference in focus.

Conventional Therapy

The focus of conventional therapy is mainly one of *anticipation*, or thinking forward. In other words, you plan your insulin according to what you anticipate your insulin needs will be over the next 6 or 12 hours. To do this, however, you must be able to predict all the factors that affect blood sugar levels—things like the food you eat and your expected level of activity. To keep everything in balance, you need to have regular eating habits and predictable levels of activity.

Is this possible? To some extent, yes. Many people are able to maintain a predictable lifestyle. You may be one of them. If so, a conventional program can give you "good to excellent" control of blood sugar. Of course, to achieve success, you must assume that everything happening to your body—your eating style, activity level, and metabolism—is similar from day to day. This assumption may be quite correct for many people with diabetes. And if so, they can use a fixed dose of insulin to achieve good control of their blood sugar.

Intensive Therapy

On the other hand, intensive therapy operates from another assumption—that your daily activity level, eating style, and metabolism are not always the same. To deal with these changes, you need to test your blood sugar frequently and vary your insulin doses accordingly. This makes the focus of intensive therapy two-pronged: (1) you anticipate your future insulin needs, and (2) you take insulin in response to both the present and future levels of your blood sugar. In essence, this type of treatment is trying to mimic two important characteristics of a normal pancreas—the ability to sense the blood sugar level and then respond with the right amount of insulin. If you have diabetes, your pancreas can no longer do this. But the goal of intensive therapy is to come close.

Who Can Benefit from Intensive Therapy?

Probably everyone who uses insulin could benefit from intensive insulin therapy, particularly in light of the new research findings of the Diabetes Control and Complications Trial (DCCT), which concluded that people who keep their blood sugar levels as close to normal as possible can reduce their risk of developing complications by 50 percent or more. In this study, that goal was accomplished using intensive therapy. The study was done only in people with Type I diabetes. However, it suggested that it was *keeping sugar levels close to normal*, not the particular insulin treatment schedule, that was most important. It also suggested that you should not lower your sugar levels so much that you have frequent or severe low blood sugar reactions, which could be dangerous. So the goal is to achieve the best level of diabetes control possible, but maintain safety!

While ultimately everyone may benefit from the intensive therapy approach, if you are new to diabetes, you may be just trying to get the basics down. You may want to use conventional therapy before trying intensive therapy. In fact, if your pancreas can still make some insulin—people with Type II and early Type I diabetes—you probably do not need intensive therapy to maintain the excellent diabetes control that the DCCT suggested was desirable.

Type I Diabetes

Some people with Type I diabetes can achieve adequate control of their blood sugar without using intensive therapy. For example, people in the early stages of Type I diabetes or during the remission ("honeymoon") stage are still able to secrete enough of their own insulin, and conventional insulin therapy may be enough. But eventually, most people with Type I diabetes lose the ability to secrete insulin altogether. And it may become necessary to use an intensive therapy program that more closely imitates the way a normal pancreas secretes insulin.

"High Goals." Many people with Type I diabetes are highly motivated to use intensive therapy. Convinced of its value in preventing complications—particularly in light of the DCCT results—they choose this approach to achieve the most normal blood sugar levels possible. Others choose intensive therapy for medical reasons, such as pregnancy or anticipated pregnancy.

BRITTLE DIABETES. For some people with Type I diabetes, their condition is so unstable that, no matter what they do, they can't even come close to gaining safe or adequate control of their blood sugar. This is often referred to as "brittle" diabetes, and intensive therapy is often an effective form of treatment. Why is blood sugar so hard to manage for some people? The answer is not always clear. But if your diabetes falls into this category, you may wish to ask your health-care team about the more precise control of intensive therapy.

LIFESTYLE CONSIDERATIONS. If you have an unpredictable lifestyle, you may also benefit from intensive therapy. Perhaps you change work shifts frequently or travel extensively. Or maybe your activity levels change hour by hour, or day to day. While these variations are not ideal, they may be unavoidable. If so, you may require a treatment program that is more adaptable to your changing routine.

Type II Diabetes

The DCCT study was done on people with Type I diabetes. Nonetheless, most experts believe its findings can be extended to people with Type II diabetes. People with Type II diabetes may also be able to reduce their risk of complications by trying to achieve normal blood sugar levels. For people with this type of diabetes, the main focus is on their meal and activity programs. Diabetes pills may be added, and insulin may be necessary for some. However, for many people with Type II diabetes, conventional therapy is often effective because the pancreas may secrete enough insulin, but it does not work as well as it should, possibly because the body's cells have developed resistance to it. In such cases, the main purpose of treatment is to provide the extra insulin the body needs to make up for this resistance.

For many people with Type II diabetes, merely "intensifying" their conventional therapy may be enough to achieve desired blood sugar goals. To do this, they would choose the conventional form of insulin treatment, such as a morning mixture of regular and intermediate insulins, presupper regular insulin and bedtime intermediate insulin. They would vary the doses somewhat when frequent blood sugar monitoring results suggest it is necessary, making their treatment more flexible and responsive.

Nonetheless, anyone who must rely on insulin injections may wish to consider intensive therapy. With this approach, the insulin dosing mimics normal blood insulin levels by providing a constant "basal" insulin level, then increasing the insulin level in response to food intake. By using such a program—closely monitoring your blood sugar and adjusting insulin accordingly—you can gain much greater control of your diabetes. In fact, the closer the insulin patterns are to normal, the more normal the blood sugar levels. And many people say they feel better.

SETTING TREATMENT GOALS

The ultimate goal of intensive therapy is precision—to achieve a more precise level of blood sugar than could be achieved with a fixed insulin dose. The DCCT study suggested that *keeping your blood sugar levels as normal as possible for as long as possible* can greatly reduce your chance of developing long-term complications from diabetes. However, the question is: Just how normal should your blood sugar levels be? Also, how much effort should be made to achieve a goal that may be reached to some extent with far less effort?

While the study suggested that you should come the closest that you safely can to normal blood sugar levels, it also made another observation. Even people with high blood sugar levels who are able to improve them somewhat, but not close to normal, are better off than they would have been with the higher levels. This means that improving your diabetes control is good for you—regardless of where you start or how much you improve! You should, of course, discuss your goals with your health-care team before making any changes in your treatment program. Remember, you will be doing most of the care yourself. You should be sure that your goals are realistic, safe and achievable.

HOW DOES INTENSIVE THERAPY WORK?

If you use intensive diabetes therapy, your insulin doses will be different from day to day, depending on your blood sugar levels at various times of the day. The doses—usually three or more per day—are varied on a daily basis. The doses are based on:

- your blood sugar level at the time of injection
- the food you recently ate and expect to eat
- your activity level, now and later

Before each meal, you perform a blood test to check your blood sugar (see Chapter 10). You then use the result of this test to determine the actual dose of insulin you need at that time, about 20 to 30 minutes before your meal, based on a "sliding scale," also called an *algorithm*. This is a treatment program that includes different insulin doses for various blood sugar levels. Examples will be given later in this chapter.

Choices of Insulin

In recent years, medical advances have made intensive therapy more feasible. New devices have made it easier to test your blood. And the new types of insulin offer a greater number of treatment options. Today, you have access to intermediate-acting insulins (NPH and Lente) and even long-acting Ultralente. These insulins can be used in a co-ordinated way with short-acting (regular) insulin to get greater control of diabetes.

Intensified Conventional Therapy—The Middle Ground

If you are looking to improve your diabetes control, it's important to approach insulin therapy as a step-by-step process. While each step may get a little more complex and involved, it will also take you a little closer to mimicking the normal pattern of a healthy pancreas. However, to jump from conventional therapy to intensive therapy would bypass a "middle ground" which might be able to get you proper control using a simpler approach than the intensive program.

For many people now using conventional insulin therapy, the first step in improving their blood sugar control is to "intensify" their present therapy. For example, if you are taking one morning injection of NPH, you may want to consider following a program of two or three fixed doses, as discussed earlier, in which you would use mixtures of regular plus intermediate-acting NPH or Lente insulin. These "mixed-dose" programs come closer than one daily injection to imitating the insulin production of a normal pancreas, which maintains a constant level of insulin (the "basal" insulin level) and then responds with additional insulin to cover food intake. That's because a mixed-dose program spreads the insulin action throughout the day, with insulin peaking at times fairly close to meals (see Figure 9-1). By using insulin more frequently—and with varying onset, peak activity, and duration—you always have some insulin in your blood.

Figure 9-1

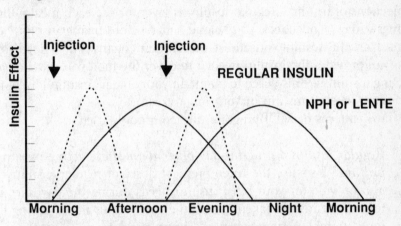

Effect of a mixed-dose insulin program for Type I diabetes: regular and intermediate insulin before breakfast and before supper.

The next step beyond using fixed doses of insulin is to vary the doses. This is done by working out a program in which more regular insulin is given in the morning and before supper if blood sugar is high, and less if it is low. This "intensified conventional" program usually uses these two daily regular injections. It is a simplified approach that is often quite successful for many people.

INTENSIVE INSULIN DOSING SCHEDULES

Most "true" intensive programs require at least three daily adjustable doses of regular insulin. Diabetes health-care experts have designed various approaches for injecting these doses. One approach is *multiple daily injections*, which involves three or more daily injections of regular insulin using standard insulin syringes. Another approach is *continuous subcutaneous insulin infusion*, commonly called the "insulin pump." The pump is a device worn outside the body that contains insulin which passes in a continuous flow from the pump through tubing and into a needle inserted under the skin. When using the pump, you test your blood sugar frequently to determine the proper insulin doses and then adjust the pump accordingly (see the discussion at end of this chapter). Let's look at both approaches in more detail.

Multiple Daily Injections (MDI)

With this method of intensive therapy, you use three or more daily injections of insulin. Regular insulin is given before each meal—three times a day. You check your blood sugar before taking insulin, and based on the result, you adjust the amount of insulin. The regular insulin provides the insulin needed to cover the food you eat. Longer-acting insulins are also used to maintain your "basal" insulin level—the constant level of insulin in your bloodstream.

Two patterns of MDI programs are commonly used:

- *Regular insulin during the day plus intermediate-acting insulin at bedtime.* Usually, the three premeal doses of regular insulin can also provide for your basal insulin needs during the daytime. Intermediate insulin taken at bedtime covers your needs during this long stretch of time when it's impractical to give injections of short-acting (regular) insulin. This program provides a great deal of flexibility. Because you are mainly using short-acting insulin during the daytime, you can adapt to any change in your activity or meal plans by adjusting your next dose of insulin.

  The program can be quite effective overnight as well. Most people have natural rises in their insulin requirements toward the end of their nighttime sleep period. For people with diabetes, this can result in rising blood sugar levels just before they awaken—"the dawn phenomenon"—if there is not enough insulin to keep the levels down. In this program, by taking an intermediate-acting insulin at bedtime, it will peak about the time that you wake up, holding the sugar levels in line at this time of day.
- *Regular plus long-acting insulin.* The other common way to provide the basal insulin supply is to use long-acting Ultralente. This insulin is usually given at breakfast and at supper, along with doses of regular insulin before each of the three meals. Ultralente is slowly absorbed, usually over a period of 24–28 hours. In some people it may last longer. When given twice a day in moderate doses (usually amounting to about half of the daily insulin dosage), it can be thought of as being essentially "peakless," providing the constant basal insulin supply that your body needs.

  This program provides a great deal of stability. In fact, Ultralente tends to smooth out the brittle patterns of some people. It also allows for more flexibility in the timing of meals. However, it is not as effective in holding "fasting" (before breakfast) sugar levels on target as the program described above that uses intermediate-acting insulin at bedtime. This is because Ultralente doesn't peak just before awakening and, therefore, doesn't counteract the "dawn phenomenon" as effectively.

NOTE: *If Ultralente and regular insulins are mixed in the same syringe, the injection should be given at once. If they are allowed to sit, some of the regular is converted into Ultralente, and the dose loses some of its immediate effect.*

Insulin Sliding Scale

People using intensive therapy will often have an *algorithm*, commonly referred to as a "sliding scale," to guide them in their adjustment of insulin doses. This is a computation that tells you how much regular insulin to take at the appropriate time of day, depending on the results of your blood sugar testing. Table 9-1 is an example of such a sliding scale.

Your physician should design a sliding scale just for you, based on your estimated insulin needs and the amount of insulin you used in the past. Then, depending on the results of your blood sugar tests, the insulin doses will be modified to help you gain maximum control of your blood sugar.

TABLE 9-1. INTENSIVE DIABETES THERAPY SLIDING SCALE

BLOOD SUGAR RANGE (MG/DL)	DOSE OF REGULAR INSULIN (UNITS)			
	BREAKFAST	PRELUNCH	PREDINNER	BEDTIME
0–50	5	4	4	0
51–100	7	5	5	0
101–150	8	6	6	0
151–200	9	6	6	0
201–250	10	7	7	0
251–300	11	8	8	0
301–400	12	9	9	0
>400	13	10	10	0

IMPORTANT NOTE: *These doses are examples. Each person must have individualized insulin doses determined by a health-care team.*

Adjusting for Low Blood Sugar

A common problem found with intensive therapy is low blood sugar. To bring it back to normal levels, follow the guidelines found in Chapter 12. Also, see the guidelines in Table 9-2.

Whenever you experience low blood sugar, you should try to determine the cause. Test your blood frequently, jotting down the results in a notebook. Also record your medication and your eating and activity schedules. You and your health-care team can often pinpoint the problem and develop a strategy to prevent low blood sugar.

Adjusting for High Blood Sugar

If you are following intensive therapy and have high blood sugar, your health-care team may advise you to make adjustments to your Ultralente or regular insulin/sliding scale doses. These may be similar to the adjustments shown in Table 9-2, but first check with your doctor to determine what's best for you.

TABLE 9-2. GUIDELINES FOR ADJUSTING ULTRALENTE AND REGULAR INSULIN/SLIDING SCALE

1. *Check for other causes*
   Before adjusting your insulin dose, you must be

   a. following your meal plan
   b. using your testing equipment correctly
   c. not sick
   d. sure you are not actually having low-blood-sugar reactions and rebounding (see the discussion of this reaction in Chapter 12)

2. *Blood sugar goals*
   Be sure you have discussed your blood sugar goals with your health-care team, and that they are safe and realistic. Generally, goals should be

   Fasting (before breakfast): 100–150 mg/dl
   Prelunch, predinner, and bedtime: 100–150 mg/dl

3. *Adjusting for high blood sugar*

   a. When fasting (prebreakfast) blood sugar is high, make the following adjustments in Ultralente insulin:

After 4 days in a row of high blood sugar tests (180 mg/dl or higher, or whatever your health-care team defines as high), verify by checking blood sugar at 2 A.M.

If the 2 A.M. blood sugar is low (less than or equal to 100 mg/dl), the high fasting test may be due to a rebound. Decrease both the morning and the evening Ultralente doses by 1 unit.

If the 2 A.M. blood sugar is high (greater than or equal to 100 mg/dl), the high fasting test may be due to insufficient insulin action overnight. Increase both the morning and the evening Ultralente doses by 1 unit.

Wait at least 4 days in between each adjustment of Ultralente. (Often, it takes even longer.)

NOTE: *If you take only 1 injection of Ultralente, adjust that dose by 1 unit as outlined above. Wait at least 4 days between each adjustment.*

b. When prelunch, predinner, or bedtime tests for blood sugar are high, adjust the regular insulin/sliding scale as follows:

For prelunch high blood sugar (180 mg/dl or higher for 3 days or whatever parameters your health-care team has given you), increase the morning scale by 1 unit.*

For predinner high blood sugar (180 mg/dl or higher for 3 days or whatever parameters your health-care team has given you), increase the lunchtime scale by 1 unit.*

For bedtime high blood sugar (180 mg/dl or higher for 3 days or whatever parameters your health-care team has given you), increase the dinner scale by 1 unit.*

Wait at least 3 days in between each adjustment in your sliding scale, unless you are having extremely high or low sugar levels.

* NOTE: *180 mg/dl or higher is a general guideline. Your health-care team may have specific guidelines for you.*

4. *Adjusting for low blood sugar*

a. If your blood sugar is low (100 mg/dl or lower, or below the lower level set for you by your health-care team) for three days in a row at the same time of day, without the symptoms of an insulin reaction or another obvious explanation, *decrease* the appropriate insulin, just as you increased the appropriate insulin in the example above. Wait two days between each adjustment in the regular insulin/sliding scale and four days between each adjustment in the Ultralente dose.

b. If you have an "unexplained" insulin reaction (blood sugar less than 60 mg/dl), which can't be explained by too little food, too much exercise, or an error in insulin dose, *decrease* the appropriate insulin *the very next day,* as noted above.

5. *Other guidelines*

a. Never adjust more than one insulin at a time.
b. Unless told otherwise, don't make more than two adjustments without calling your doctor or nurse educator.
c. To improve the absorption of Ultralente, you may need to use different injection sites for the morning and evening injections. The members of your health-care team will discuss this with you if they feel it is necessary.
d. Check your weight. It is very easy to gain weight using this or any form of intensive insulin therapy. If you do gain weight, review your meal plan with your dietitian.
e. Snacks: There generally is no need to snack on this regimen. But if your bedtime blood sugar is less than 200 mg/dl, you may need a snack to prevent a reaction overnight. You may also need to snack before or after exercise.
f. Your insulin can lose its stability (weaken) if left out of the refrigerator for too long a period. Do not leave it out of the refrigerator for more than 30 days. Bottles currently in use should not be exposed to temperatures greater than 75°. Extra bottles of insulin should be refrigerated.

THE INSULIN INFUSION PUMP

One of the great advances in diabetes therapy in recent years is the development of the insulin infusion pump. This is a device that "pumps" the required amount of insulin into the body. Currently, only a manually adjusted pump is available. It is worn on the outside of the body and releases insulin to the tissues of the body by way of tubing and a needle. The person using the pump must determine the proper insulin dose by testing his or her blood sugar, similar to the way multiple daily injections programs work. The dose is adjusted based on the test results.

Infusion pumps use only regular insulin. They mimic the pancreas's secretion of insulin by providing a slow, constant flow of insulin through the tubing and needle—the "basal" insulin supply. They also provide the insulin needed to cover incoming food. These additional doses of insulin are called *boluses*, the amount of which is determined by using a sliding scale similar to that used to determine regular insulin doses in MDI programs (see above).

Note that these pumps pump insulin into the body continuously. For this reason, users must test their blood sugar often to ensure the device is being used safely and effectively. Only with frequent blood testing can they make a proper decision about the flow of insulin. Researchers are trying to develop an automatic pump that would be implanted in the body. Ideally, this system would measure the blood sugar level by itself, then inject the correct amount of insulin automatically. The user would not have to do regular blood testing or make adjustments to the pump. Scientists hope this system will be available soon.

Injections or Pump?

If you decide on intensive insulin therapy, you have two basic options—multiple daily injections or the insulin pump. At first glance, the pump may look easier to use. But there are several factors to consider.

Compared with a simple syringe, the pump is part of a more complex system, and it requires more frequent blood testing. In addition, insulin is continuously being infused into the body with the pump. If proper caution is not exercised, the risks of using a pump can be greater than those associated with injection. Therefore, the decision to use pump therapy should not be taken lightly.

Yet for people who make the decision to use a pump and do everything that is necessary to manage this approach, successful control often results. Pumps come the closest to mimicking normal insulin patterns, so they can come the closest to providing normal blood sugar levels. Also, with the smoother insulin patterns, users often report that they feel better.

Too many people make the mistake of thinking that a pump will allow them to abandon the other parts of their diabetes program, such as meal planning and exercise. This is not true. They remain an essential part of your program. So, in accordance with the step-by-step approach discussed earlier, most people start with multiple daily injections. Only if that is not satisfactory do they consider using a pump.

NUTRITION AND INTENSIVE THERAPY

Intensive therapy for diabetes is not new. What *is* new are the several ways you can manage your treatment program through nutrition, many of which have been previously discussed in Chapters 3 and 4. Below are four meal-plan options that you can discuss with your health-care team to help you with your intensive therapy:

- *Food choices.* This method is specifically designed to simplify meal planning, yet still maintain consistency in your food intake (see Appendix: Food Choice Lists).
- *Exchanges.* This system is the most commonly used meal planning technique. It allows you to choose from six food groups. Within each group, you may make substitutions while still maintaining proper amounts of nutrients (see Chapter 3).
- *Carbohydrate counting.* In this method, you count all the carbohydrates that you eat. Your dietitian can show you how to use this method. See discussion in Chapter 3.
- *Total available glucose* (TAG). This is a very complex system based on the available amount of glucose from certain nutrients.

There are pros and cons to all the foregoing methods. Be sure to discuss the various options with your health-care team, who will help tailor a program to best fit your individual needs.

WHAT'S BEST FOR YOU?

There are many ways to use insulin, and you should work with your health-care team to identify the best program for you. Remember, the overall goal is to create a dosing schedule that works in concert with your meal plan and exercise. Not everyone can manage intensive diabetes therapy. But research now shows what experts at the Joslin Diabetes Center have been saying to their patients for nearly a century—if you keep your blood sugar as close to normal as possible, you can decrease your risk of complications.

If intensive therapy is the best plan for you, it will take some effort to develop an effective routine. You will have to closely monitor your blood sugar. In addition, you will need the support of a skilled health-care team. Intensive therapy is not a "solo act," and the information in this chapter only broadly covers the details of such a program. Intensive therapy shouldn't be tried by people who are not trained in its techniques. Furthermore, the results of intensive therapy may take some time to achieve. It often takes months to get the program working just right. In fact, your reward may be what *doesn't* happen, rather than what does. For example, your program may help you prevent a severe insulin reaction (low blood sugar). Or it may be that your reward will come even further into the future—the reduced risk of developing complications from diabetes that everyone is trying to avoid. But whether your rewards are now or in the future, they can be great. And the feeling of success and good health can make the effort all worthwhile.

For more detailed information on how to embark on intensive diabetes therapy, see Richard Beaser's *Outsmarting Diabetes* (published by Chronimed, Inc., Minneapolis, 1994).

Part Four

MONITORING AND ADJUSTING YOUR TREATMENT PROGRAM

CHAPTER 10

Monitoring Your Diabetes

IF YOU HAVE DIABETES, your body's metabolism is no longer on "automatic." Without help, it can no longer keep your blood sugar in normal range. That's where you play a key role—stepping in on behalf of your body to make decisions about your treatment. To do that, you need to know your blood sugar levels. And that can be done by testing your blood on a regular schedule, or "monitoring."

You stand to gain many benefits from monitoring. It will help keep your blood sugar in control. You will feel better and have more energy to carry out your daily activities with enthusiasm. Your life, both at home and at work, will be interrupted by fewer problems related to diabetes. If you use your monitoring results to make adjustments in your diabetes treatment program to get your blood sugar under better control, you are less likely to develop long-term complications.

Don't be fooled into thinking that monitoring isn't necessary. You may decide, for example, "Since I'm not having any symptoms of high or low blood sugar, why bother with all of this monitoring?" Or you may be tempted to think, "Since home monitoring meters aren't quite as accurate as those used in my doctor's lab, my results aren't useful." Such thinking is flawed. Just because you feel okay doesn't necessarily mean you are meeting your treatment goals. The fact is you usually will not have symptoms when your blood sugar is moderately out of control. As for your home testing, the degree of accuracy that a good meter can provide is close enough to professional results. It will give you very useful information to care for your diabetes.

The best plan is to use a monitoring system that detects high or low blood sugars *long before symptoms appear.* That way, when high or low blood sugars occasionally do occur, you will be ready to adjust your food, exercise, and medications to get things under control.

How to Monitor Your Diabetes

You can monitor your diabetes in two basic ways—by testing urine and by testing blood. Before the late 1970s, the only way that people with diabetes could monitor their own condition was by measuring the amount of sugar in their urine. The test was done by dipping specially treated strips into the urine, which would change color, depending on the level of sugar in the urine. Such tests were not very accurate, however, and a precise measurement only could be made through blood tests available in a doctor's office or hospital laboratory.

During the late 1970s, however, medical technology created a new way to measure diabetes control—home blood sugar monitoring. Because the test is simple to perform and can be done at home, it has been a significant breakthrough, providing more precise results than urine testing ever could.

Testing Urine for Sugar—A Bygone Era

To understand how urine testing works—and why it is no longer recommended for monitoring diabetes—it's important to review how your body obtains and uses blood sugar. Your digestive system changes the carbohydrates in the food you eat into the form of sugar called glucose, which is absorbed into the blood. With the help of insulin, your cells use the sugar for energy or store it for future use. When enough insulin is available and when the body can use it properly, blood sugar levels are maintained within the normal range of 60–140 mg/dl.

Figure 10-1 shows how blood sugar can be maintained at normal levels throughout the day *when sufficient insulin is available and used properly.* Notice how the blood sugar rises soon after eating—always staying within normal levels—and then falls back as insulin processes the sugar from the food. Before you had diabetes, your pancreas was able to do this automatically by secreting the necessary amount of insulin to keep your blood sugar in normal range no matter what or how much you ate.

Now that you have diabetes, your pancreas is unable to keep up with

Figure 10-1
Normal Metabolism

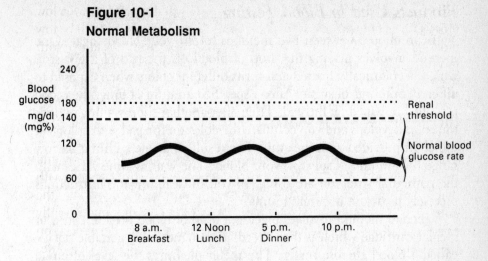

your insulin needs and sugar builds up in the bloodstream. The level can get so high that your kidneys can't recycle sugar back into the bloodstream and it eventually "spills" over into the urine. However, this does not happen until your blood sugar is *well above the desired level*. For this reason, health-care professionals recommend that you test your blood, rather than your urine. You'll be able to detect high blood sugar before it reaches the "renal (kidney) threshold" and spills over into the urine.

TESTING BLOOD FOR SUGAR . . . THE BEST APPROACH

Blood testing is the best approach to finding out how well you are controlling your diabetes. To test the level of sugar in your blood, you must first obtain a drop of blood by pricking one of your fingers. This can be done with a sterile *lancet*, a special type of needle used only for this purpose. A good place to prick is the side of the finger, near the tip. Compared with the center of the finger, the side has fewer nerve endings to cause pain. Also, more blood is available.

While some people prick themselves using the lancet alone, without using a device, many prefer using a finger-pricking device. There are a number of instruments developed by different companies for this purpose, all of which hold a lancet activated by a spring. Most of the devices come equipped with various sizes of "guards" or "platforms" used to adjust the depth that the lancet enters the skin. That way, you won't penetrate the skin too deeply.

Products Used in Blood Testing

You can choose between two methods to test your blood sugar. One method involves placing the drop of blood on the pad of a test strip which is chemically treated and turns different colors when exposed to different amounts of sugar. After a specified amount of time, the blood is blotted or wiped off the pad. Then after another short waiting period, the color develops and you compare the color on the pad with colors on the chart provided with the strip. The results indicate within a narrow range the amount of sugar in your blood. The waiting time varies with the particular strip you are using, so you must follow the instructions precisely to obtain accurate results.

A second method involves placing a drop of blood on a test strip or special cartridge which is then "read" by a hand-held, portable device called a blood glucose meter. The meter measures the level of blood sugar and displays it on a screen. Some devices can store the results of a large number of tests in a computer memory and provide you with a printed readout of the results. Your doctor or nurse educator will help you choose the best method of blood testing for your situation. They will also help you choose a specific type of test strip and meter and teach you how to use it.

Always follow the procedures carefully. The results will not be accurate if your technique is faulty. One common error is not applying enough blood onto the test pad; it is essential to use a large drop of blood. Other mistakes include incomplete coverage of the pad, incomplete wiping of the blood from the pad, incorrect timing of the test, and failure to clean the meter. Improper handling or storage of the test strips or meters also may lead to errors. Strips for blood testing should be kept in a cool, dry place and discarded after the expiration date shown on the container.

You can also get inaccurate results by using a faulty meter, so be sure to regularly check your equipment and technique. This is done by doing a self-test with your equipment at the same time that a lab test is done. You then compare the results. If you use the test strips, your reading should be within 20 percent of the lab results. If you use a meter, your reading should be within 10 to 15 percent. Special glucose "control solutions" are also available to check the meters. Use them as directed by the manufacturer.

Keeping Track of Test Results

For people who do not have diabetes, the normal blood sugar level before breakfast is under 115 mg/dl. The normal level at other times— before other meals or two hours after eating—is less than 140 mg/dl. The acceptable range for someone with diabetes may be slightly higher, so your physician may establish different goals for you. Blood testing tells you fairly accurately what your blood sugar level is at a particular time. It can detect high, low, or normal levels, and thus allow you to monitor your blood sugar patterns throughout the day and night and make proper adjustments.

Proper record keeping is a crucial part of this process. A log or record book provides space to enter your blood sugar levels at particular times of day for a number of days running. There is also space to record your insulin doses at particular times of each day, and a column in which to note any significant events of the day such as changes in activity, food consumption or timing, and hypoglycemic reactions (low blood sugar). (See the Diabetes Monitoring Record in Figure 10-2.) Using this record, you and your health-care team can more accurately determine proper insulin doses, adjustments in your diabetes pills, and changes to your meal and exercise regimen.

Testing for Hemoglobin A_1 and A_{1c}

In addition to testing your blood for glucose, your physician may want to monitor your diabetes with a relatively new test that measures total *glycosylated hemoglobin*, also called the *hemoglobin A_1 or A_{1C}*. This test provides information that helps to assess your average blood sugar level over a period of approximately eight weeks. To obtain this information, your physician will take a sample of your blood and send it to a laboratory for testing.

The basis for the test lies in the way blood sugar interacts with hemoglobin. Hemoglobin is a substance that carries oxygen from the lungs to all parts of the body; it also removes carbon dioxide. Hemoglobin is found in the red cells of the blood, which have a life span of four months. As old cells die, your body constantly creates new ones. Most of the hemoglobin in the red blood cells is called hemoglobin A. Normally, a small amount of hemoglobin A exists in a slightly different form called hemoglobin A_1. It is formed when blood sugar attaches to the hemoglobin in the red blood cells.

The amount of sugar that becomes attached to the hemoglobin de-

FIGURE 10-2. DIABETES MONITORING RECORD

Patient's Full Name _____

Street _____

City & State _____

Date 19	Glucose Test Results					Insulin								Comments
	Before Break-fast	Before Noon Meal	Before Supper	At Bedtime	Other	Before Breakfast		Before Lunch	Before Supper		Bedtime			
						Reg.	Long/Inter.	Reg.	Reg.	Long/Inter.	Reg.	Long/Inter.		

Key: Reg. = Regular or Clear Insulin
Inter. = Intermediate-acting insulin: NPH or Lente
Long = Long-acting insulin: Ultralente

In "Comments" section above record variations in activity, food consumption, or timing, and hypoglycemic reactions.

General Comments: _____

_____

_____

Physician/Nurse Educator: _____

pends on the amount of sugar in the blood. This attachment occurs very slowly. If you experience a sudden, brief rise in blood sugar, there is little effect on the amount of sugar that becomes permanently attached. However, high levels of blood sugar sustained over a period of several weeks will attach to the hemoglobin. This will show up in a test for hemoglobin A_1, and reflects the average of your glucose control over the past 2–3 months.

Labs use different methods to measure hemoglobin A_1. The normal ranges vary according to the method used, so the results of one method cannot be compared with those of another. Whenever you are interpreting the results of a test, be sure to check which method is being used and the appropriate normal range. In the method used at the Joslin Diabetes Center to measure hemoglobin A_{1C}, the reading for affected red blood cells ranges from 4 to 6 percent when blood sugar levels are consistently normal. When blood sugar levels are very high over a period of time, the level may reach 16 percent or more. Some laboratories measure hemoglobin A_1, of which hemoglobin A_{1C} is a portion. When this method is used, the normal range is approximately 5.4 to 7.4 percent.

It is important to note, however, that in interpreting tests for hemoglobin A_1, near-normal results don't necessarily mean that you have maintained acceptable blood sugar levels on a day-to-day basis. In fact, a satisfactory reading may actually reflect the average of some very high and very low blood sugar levels during the eight-week period. In such cases, the amount of sugar that becomes attached to the hemoglobin could be similar to readings obtained when blood sugar is consistently closer to normal. You could be getting a distorted view of what has really occurred.

For that reason, the test for hemoglobin A_{1C} alone doesn't give the whole picture of whether you are adequately managing your diabetes properly. But used in conjunction with test results from regular monitoring of the blood, the A_{1C} test does provide useful information that may detect if something is amiss in your treatment program. For example, if you show consistently acceptable results from regular monitoring but a high hemoglobin A_{1C}, you may need to monitor your blood more frequently to detect fluctuations that may occur at times of the day you are not monitoring.

Another possibility is that there is something wrong with the way you are doing the regular tests for blood sugar. In that case, you should check with your physician or nurse educator to correct your technique.

WHEN TO MONITOR YOUR DIABETES

There is no single monitoring schedule that is appropriate for every person with diabetes. How often you monitor your diabetes depends, in part, on the type of diabetes you have, the medications you take, and when you take them.

If You Use Insulin

If you use insulin, you will monitor at times that are related to the action pattern of your medication. Following are examples of how to monitor two mixed doses of insulin and a single dose of intermediate-acting insulin.

TWO MIXED DOSES OF INSULIN. If you have Type I diabetes, you may require at least two injections a day once your body is making little or no insulin. Each injection may consist of a mixture of short- and intermediate-acting insulins. One injection is given before breakfast, and the other before dinner. Some people with Type II diabetes may also have a similar injection schedule.

If this is your schedule, your physician may want you to monitor your diabetes by testing your blood four times a day. The best times are before breakfast, lunch, dinner, and at bedtime before your evening snack. In testing this way, you can assess how well the different insulins are working to maintain near-normal blood sugar. Below are guidelines to interpret those tests:

- *Before-breakfast test.* Shows if the dose of intermediate-acting insulin you injected the previous day before dinner has maintained satisfactory blood sugar levels throughout the night.
- *Before-lunch test.* Indicates if the short-acting insulin injected before breakfast is adequate for the period between breakfast and lunch.
- *Before-dinner test.* Shows if the intermediate-acting insulin injected before breakfast is adequate for the period between lunch and dinner.
- *Before-bedtime test.* Indicates if the short-acting insulin injected before the evening meal is adequate for the period between dinner and bedtime.

SINGLE DOSE OF INTERMEDIATE-ACTING INSULIN. Some people with Type II diabetes may be managing their condition with a single dose of intermediate-acting insulin before breakfast. If this is your schedule, you may not have to monitor as frequently as people using two mixed doses. Testing before breakfast and dinner may be sufficient. Here are some ways to interpret those tests:

- *Before-breakfast test*. Shows if you maintained satisfactory blood sugar levels throughout the previous night.
- *Before-dinner test*. Indicates if the intermediate-acting insulin injected before breakfast is adequate for the daytime hours.

If your treatment program includes a dose of intermediate-acting insulin before dinner, you should monitor your blood sugar several times a month between 2 and 3 A.M. Plan to do this whether you have Type I or Type II diabetes. The tests will indicate the effect of the predinner insulin on your blood sugar in the middle of the night— when the insulin activity is at its peak. This test is very important, because your blood sugar could drop very low without awakening you.

There are many other patterns of insulin treatment. Your health-care team can tell you which testing schedule will be best for your particular treatment program. And remember, always record the test results. Keeping track of the results of your monitoring is very important to gauge the effectiveness of your treatment program.

If You Do Not Use Insulin

If you have Type II diabetes and do not use insulin, you may be asked to monitor once or twice a day. Such a schedule would provide the following information:

- *Before-breakfast test*. Indicates if the insulin supplied by your body was sufficient to maintain satisfactory blood sugar levels throughout the previous night.
- *After-dinner test*. Shows if the insulin supplied by your body is sufficient to lower the blood sugar levels that naturally rise after your evening meal.

You also may be asked to monitor more frequently, particularly if you are just embarking on a treatment plan, are starting a new exercise program, are beginning a new oral agent, or have other circumstances that might require more frequent monitoring.

MONITORING KETONES

At certain times, it is very important to test your urine for substances called ketones. This is particularly true if you are sick, when you have a greater chance of developing extremely high levels of blood sugar (see Chapter 13). Whenever this happens, your body starts to burn fatty acids. This leads to the production of ketones, which in the presence of high blood sugar can cause a medical emergency. Another time to test for ketones is when you are planning to exercise (discussed in Chapter 5). If your blood sugar is above 240 mg/dl, you should test for ketones. If ketones are present, do not exercise until the source of the problem has been found and corrected.

There are three products on the market for monitoring your urine for ketones: Acetest, Ketostix, and Chemstrip K. All of the tests are simple to perform and provide accurate results. You can buy them at your pharmacy without a prescription. Your health-care team will help you choose the most appropriate product.

Acetest involves placing a drop of urine on a tablet and observing the change in color of the tablet. The color is then compared with colors on a color chart supplied with the product. Ketostix and Chemstrip K consist of test strips similar to those used for monitoring blood for sugar. Directions are provided with each of the products. Follow them carefully. Correct timing is very important.

OVERALL BENEFITS OF MONITORING

Using the information gathered from monitoring, you can detect single instances of high or low blood sugar. If you use insulin, single episodes can be caused by drawing up and injecting an incorrect amount of insulin. They can also be caused by eating too much or too little food, or by a sudden change in activity. Whenever single incidents occur, you should try to determine the cause and find a way to prevent the same thing from happening again.

Monitoring can also show patterns of consistently high or low blood sugar that are occurring at the same time each day over a period of days.

When this happens, your health-care team may suggest a change in your meal plan, type or timing of exercise, or a change in your medication (insulin or diabetes pills). They may also ask you to monitor more frequently to discover what is happening with your blood sugar levels at different times of the day. Once your diabetes is well managed, you may be able to reduce the schedule.

If you are following "intensive diabetes therapy," the basic idea behind that form of treatment revolves around closely monitoring your blood sugar and making adjustments in your diet, exercise, and insulin. In this type of therapy, you will be asked to monitor your blood sugar frequently, perhaps 4 to 6 times a day. Whatever your form of treatment, the rewards of monitoring can be great. As always, your goal is to keep your blood sugar at near-normal levels at all times, to feel better and to help prevent long-term complications of diabetes.

CHAPTER 11

Adjusting for High Blood Sugar

DESPITE YOUR BEST INTENTIONS, not every day will go smoothly in your treatment program. As you monitor your blood sugar, don't be surprised if you occasionally find that your levels are too high or low. This can happen even if your diabetes is well managed. Your goal is to have as few episodes as possible and to treat them while the symptoms are mild. By learning the early signs of high and low blood sugar, you can make the proper adjustments before more serious problems develop.

WHAT IS HIGH BLOOD SUGAR?

When monitoring your blood sugar, you should always record and analyze the results. Your blood sugar is generally considered high when it is *180 mg/dl or higher at the same time of day for three days in a row.* However, during periods of time that you are adjusting your insulin doses, different target levels may be set or longer periods of time may be indicated before action is taken.

Symptoms of High Blood Sugar

Many people with high blood sugar often don't experience any obvious physical symptoms that alert them that their blood sugar is too high. On the other hand, some people may experience symptoms similar to those which led them to discover they have diabetes, such as thirst, fatigue, or blurred vision. With or without symptoms, the best way to tell if you have high blood sugar is through monitoring. Only by regularly testing your blood will you get a good idea of your blood sugar levels.

Causes of High Blood Sugar

Your treatment program is based on a delicate balance of food intake, exercise, and medications. The most frequent cause of high blood sugar is too much food. If you eat too much—more food than outlined in your meal plan—the amount of sugar in your blood will exceed what was planned. The amount of exercise and medication prescribed to offset your meal plan will be inadequate to help your body convert the food into energy. Excess glucose may build up in your blood, resulting in high blood sugar.

A second cause of high blood sugar is not getting the amount of exercise planned in your treatment program. Exercise lowers the amount of sugar in your blood, and if you don't exercise as much as was planned in your treatment program, your blood sugar may rise. And finally, high blood sugar can also be caused by having too little insulin in your bloodstream or by your cells resisting the action of insulin. Below are guidelines for what to do in these situations.

Adjusting Diabetes Pills

If you have Type II diabetes, your pancreas can still produce insulin. But it may not be enough or efficient enough to maintain blood sugar within a normal range—even if you have achieved a proper weight and are following your exercise and meal plans. In such cases, your doctor may prescribe diabetes pills to boost your body's production of insulin. Or after getting the advice of your health-care team, you may need to begin taking insulin. So if your blood sugar is running consistently high, call your doctor to discuss whether you should begin or increase your diabetes pills or perhaps should begin taking insulin.

Adjusting Insulin

If you take insulin and your blood sugar levels are high, your physician may recommend adjusting your insulin dose. But before doing so, be sure there are no other explanations for the high test results. Did you eat extra food or snacks? Did you change your activity level? Did you make mistakes in measuring or timing your present insulin dose? Did you inject into an area of skin where absorption is poor? Have you gained weight? Or perhaps you are using new prescriptions or over-the-counter drugs that may be increasing your blood sugar (see Chapter 21 for further discussion of this topic). If you answered "yes" to any of these questions, you should follow your present treatment program more carefully, rather than increasing your insulin dose. If you answered "no," you probably need more insulin.

The guidelines for adjusting insulin for high blood sugar depend on many factors: the peak activity of the insulins you are using, the times of day the injections are given, and the times your blood sugar is high. If your blood sugar is high after a particular insulin reaches its peak activity, you probably need to adjust that insulin. Let's say, for example, you use a mixed dose of short- and intermediate-acting insulin before breakfast, with the intermediate-acting insulin reaching its peak activity in midafternoon. If your before-dinner test shows high blood sugar, you may need additional intermediate-acting insulin in that mixed dose.

General guidelines for adjusting insulin when blood sugar is high are listed below, followed by specific ways to handle the various types of insulins. Always check with your health-care team before following these guidelines. Your doctor may recommend a slightly different approach. Please note that these guidelines are *for days when you feel well,* even though your tests for blood sugar are high. Note, too, that your health-care team may provide other instructions that apply specifically to you, especially if you are using a form of "intensive diabetes therapy." Also be sure to note the "special circumstances" category.

GENERAL GUIDELINES

Follow these guidelines on days you are well:

- If two or more of the blood sugar tests done each day are high for three days in a row, adjust for the "high" test that occurs earliest in the day. Do not adjust more than one dose or type of insulin at a time, unless directed by your health-care team.
- After adjusting your dose, wait three days for your blood sugar level to improve. If there is no improvement, make another adjustment

to that same dose. Do not adjust your insulin a third time without consulting your doctor.
- Never increase the before-dinner or bedtime dose of intermediate-acting insulin without also testing between 2 and 3 A.M. for low blood sugar during the night, a condition discussed in Chapter 12.
- Never increase an insulin dose until you are sure the high blood sugar is not caused by a "rebound," a condition also discussed in Chapter 12.
- Unless your doctor advises you to do otherwise, do not reduce your insulin dose unless you are having insulin reactions (symptoms of low blood sugar). See Chapter 12 for further instructions.

SPECIAL CIRCUMSTANCES

Follow these guidelines under the special circumstances described below:

- If your blood sugar is 240 mg/dl, check for ketones in the urine. If ketones are present, call your doctor or nurse educator immediately.
- If your blood sugar is 400 mg/dl or higher, call your physician or nurse educator immediately, even if ketones are not present.
- If your blood sugar is 240 mg/dl or higher, and you are sick, follow the sick-day guidelines in Chapter 13.

SPECIFIC GUIDELINES

Remember, except for emergencies, you should first check with your health-care team before using the specific guidelines outlined below. They may wish to adapt them to your particular needs.

When adjusting your insulin for high blood sugar, follow the instructions in the section below that relates to the type of insulin you take and when you take it.

Intermediate-acting insulin (NPH or Lente) taken before breakfast:

1. *If your blood sugar before dinner is, for three days in a row, higher than the level set by your physician:*
   —and your present dose is less than 10 units, increase the insulin dose by 1 unit on the morning of the fourth day.

—and your present dose is 10 units or more, increase the insulin by 2 units on the morning of the fourth day.

2. *If your blood sugar before breakfast, lunch, or bedtime is higher than the level set by your physician but is acceptable before dinner:*
—call your physician. You may need other doses of insulin.

Short-acting (regular) and intermediate-acting insulin (NPH or Lente) taken before breakfast:

1. *If your blood sugar before lunch is, for three days in a row, higher than the level set by your physician:*
—and your present dose is less than 10 units, increase the amount of regular insulin by 1 unit on the morning of the fourth day.
—and your present dose is 10 units or more, increase the amount of regular insulin by 2 units on the morning of the fourth day.
2. *If your blood sugar before dinner is, for three days in a row, higher than the level set by your physician:*
—and your present dose is less than 10 units, increase the amount of NPH or Lente insulin by 1 unit on the morning of the fourth day.
—and your present dose is 10 units or more, increase the amount of NPH or Lente insulin by 2 units on the morning of the fourth day.
3. *If your blood sugar before breakfast or bedtime is, for three days in a row, higher than the level set by your physician but acceptable before dinner:*
—call your physician. You may need an evening dose of insulin.

Intermediate-acting insulin (NPH or Lente) taken before breakfast and again before dinner or bedtime:

1. *If your blood sugar before breakfast is, for three days in a row, higher than the level set by your physician, check for "rebound" by testing your blood sugar between 2 and 3 A.M. the next morning. If rebound is ruled out:*
—and your present dose is less than 10 units, increase the amount of NPH or Lente insulin by 1 unit in your next evening dose.
—and your present dose is 10 units or more, increase the amount of NPH or Lente insulin by 2 units in your next evening dose.

2. *If your blood sugar before lunch or bedtime is, for three days in a row, higher than the level set by your physician but acceptable before breakfast:*
   —call your physician. You may need short-acting insulin.
3. *If your blood sugar before dinner is, for three days in a row, higher than the level set by your physician:*
   —and your present dose is less than 10 units, increase the amount of NPH or Lente insulin by 1 unit on the morning of the fourth day.
   —and your present dose is 10 units or more, increase the amount of NPH or Lente insulin by 2 units on the morning of the fourth day.

Short-acting (regular) and intermediate-acting insulin (NPH or Lente) before breakfast and intermediate-acting insulin (NPH or Lente) before dinner or bedtime:

1. *If your blood sugar before breakfast is, for three days in a row, higher than the level set by your physician, check for "rebound" by testing your blood sugar between 2 and 3 A.M. the next morning. If rebound is ruled out:*
   —and your present dose is less than 10 units, increase the amount of NPH or Lente insulin by 1 unit in your next evening dose.
   —and your present dose is 10 units or more, increase the amount of NPH or Lente insulin by 2 units in your next evening dose.
2. *If your blood sugar before lunch is, for three days in a row, higher than the level set by your physician:*
   —and your present dose is less than 10 units, increase the amount of regular insulin by 1 unit on the morning of the fourth day.
   —and your present dose is 10 units or more, increase the amount of regular insulin by 2 units on the morning of the fourth day.
3. *If your blood sugar before dinner is, for three days in a row, higher than the level set by your physician:*
   —and your present dose is less than 10 units, increase the amount of NPH or Lente insulin by 1 unit on the morning of the fourth day.
   —and your present dose is 10 units or more, increase the amount of NPH or Lente insulin by 2 units on the morning of the fourth day.

4. *If your blood sugar before bedtime is, for three days in a row, higher than the level set by your physician, but all other tests are acceptable:*
—call your physician. You may need a short-acting insulin before dinner.

Short-acting (regular) and intermediate-acting insulin (NPH or Lente) before breakfast, short-acting (regular) before dinner, and intermediate-acting (NPH or Lente) at bedtime:

1. *If your blood sugar before breakfast is, for three days in a row, higher than the level set by your physician, check for "rebound" by testing your blood sugar between 2 and 3 A.M. the next morning. If rebound is ruled out:*
—and your present evening dose is less than 10 units, increase the amount of NPH or Lente insulin by 1 unit in your next bedtime dose.
—and your present evening dose is 10 units or more, increase the amount of NPH or Lente insulin by 2 units in your next bedtime dose.
2. *If your blood sugar before lunch is, for three days in a row, higher than the level set by your physician:*
—and your present morning dose is less than 10 units, increase the amount of regular insulin by 1 unit on the morning of the fourth day.
—and your present morning dose is 10 units or more, increase the amount of regular insulin by 2 units on the morning of the fourth day.
3. *If your blood sugar before dinner is, for three days in a row, higher than the level set by your physician:*
—and your present morning dose is less than 10 units, increase the amount of regular insulin by 1 unit on the morning of the fourth day.
—and your present morning dose is 10 units or more, increase the amount of regular insulin by 2 units on the morning of the fourth day.
4. *If your blood sugar before bedtime is, for three days in a row, higher than the level set by your physician:*
—and your present before-dinner dose is less than 10 units, increase the amount of regular insulin by 1 unit before dinner on the fourth day.

—and your present before-dinner dose is 10 units or more, increase the amount of regular insulin by 2 units before dinner on the fourth day.

If, for any of the aforementioned treatment programs, you discover that your blood sugar level drops too low during the night, reduce the evening NPH or Lente insulin (or morning, if that is all you take) and contact your health-care team to talk about adjusting your program.

Special Instructions for People Who Use Ultralente

If you use Ultralente as part of "intensive diabetes therapy," please refer to the guidelines on pages 138–140 of Chapter 9.

EXTREME SITUATIONS

Whenever you have extremely high levels of blood sugar, you and the people you live with must be prepared to act. Left untreated, this situation could result in coma or death.

Ketoacidosis

Serious problems may occur if your blood sugar gets so high that your body turns to its fat stores for energy, leading to the production of ketones, which build up in the blood and spill into the urine. This is more likely in people who have Type I diabetes (insulin-dependent). But it also can occur in some people who have Type II diabetes (non-insulin-dependent), although it is much less likely.

Allowed to go untreated, the combination of high blood sugar and ketones can lead to *ketoacidosis*, a serious and life-threatening condition. Ketoacidosis does not happen suddenly, but rather develops over a period of days if blood sugar levels remain untreated. Ketoacidosis is a medical emergency. Symptoms of ketoacidosis include nausea, stomach pain, vomiting, chest pain, rapid shallow breathing, and difficulty staying awake.

On days when you're sick, you are at a much greater risk for ketoacidosis. That's why it is vital that you follow the guidelines for sick-day care in Chapter 13 any time you are experiencing illness or other situations associated with severe stress. By following these instructions, you will prevent your blood sugar and ketone levels from rising to a point where they cause ketoacidosis.

Hyperosmolar-Nonketotic Coma

Another serious problem that can result from high blood sugar is *hyperosmolar-nonketotic coma*. This condition occurs in people with Type II diabetes when the blood sugar is so high that the body becomes dehydrated, causing a severe imbalance in the body's chemistry. Hyperosmolar-nonketotic coma is most common in older patients. Like ketoacidosis, it develops over a period of days as a result of untreated high blood sugar, illness, or dehydration.

Symptoms of the onset of hyperosmolar-nonketotic coma include excessive thirst or urination, increased hunger, drowsiness, nausea or vomiting, abdominal pain, and rapid shallow breathing. Similar to ketoacidosis, you are at a higher risk of hyperosmolar-nonketotic coma when you are sick. Be sure to read Chapter 13 to learn how to prevent this problem.

WHAT TO DO IN EMERGENCY SITUATIONS

If coma or unconsciousness occurs from high blood sugar, you will need immediate emergency attention. You should be taken by ambulance to a hospital.

Be sure that people at home or work know what to do in the event of an emergency. Also, whenever you are sick, ask someone to check on you. And at all times, wear an identification tag that says you have diabetes.

SUMMARY

What to do when you experience the symptoms of high blood sugar:

1. Test your blood sugar to make sure that it's high. Compare your blood sugar level with the level set by your doctor.
2. Follow your diabetes treatment plan. Eat your meals and snacks as advised by your health-care team. Do the same amount of

physical activity or exercise every day. Check your blood sugar level.

3. If you take diabetes pills, take the prescribed amount at the correct time.
4. If you use insulin, adjust it according to your doctor's directions.
5. Call your doctor if your blood sugar is over 180 mg/dl for 3 days in a row, or if you are sick.

CHAPTER 12

Adjusting for Low Blood Sugar

I<small>N TREATING DIABETES</small>, we usually think of trying to control *high* blood sugar. But at times, people with diabetes can actually experience *low* blood sugar, also called hypoglycemia. Low blood sugar is more likely to occur in people who use insulin, so most of the guidelines outlined below apply to this group of people. However, low blood sugar also may occur in people who use diabetes pills to treat their condition, so some of the guidelines—particularly those relating to diet and exercise—might also apply. And remember, these guidelines will help you treat low blood sugar on *days you are well.* For days you are sick, please see the guidelines in Chapter 13.

W<small>HAT</small> I<small>S</small> L<small>OW</small> B<small>LOOD</small> S<small>UGAR</small>?

If your blood sugar is below 60 mg/dl, you have "low blood sugar." You can often tell if your blood sugar is low simply by the way you feel. But it's important to be sure. *Always* confirm the condition by testing your blood.

Symptoms of Low Blood Sugar

Low blood sugar can occur suddenly. Early signs include shakiness, nervousness, sweating, dizziness, weakness, irritability, hunger, and heart pounding. Symptoms that occur more slowly include crying, anger, drowsiness, confusion, staggered gait, inability to complete work, blurred vision, and headache.

Whenever you feel any of these symptoms coming on, you should test your blood immediately, if possible. Testing is important because some of the symptoms of low blood sugar are similar to those of other medical conditions unrelated to diabetes. Also, be aware that some people who have had diabetes for a long time or who control their diabetes very tightly may lose the ability to recognize some of the symptoms. In such cases, extra caution—and blood monitoring—is very important.

If your blood sugar is low, you should begin treatment right away. If you allow it to go untreated, more serious problems may develop, such as convulsions or unconsciousness. At the end of this chapter, you will learn what to do in such cases.

People with Type II diabetes (non-insulin-dependent) are much less likely to experience low blood sugar levels, especially reactions that would leave them unconscious.

Causes of Low Blood Sugar

The most common cause of low blood sugar is poor timing of meals or snacks. Anytime you reduce the amount of food you eat, or skip or delay a meal, you will have less sugar in your blood than if you had remained true to your meal plan. This creates a situation in which your body has too much insulin for the amount of sugar in your blood. The insulin works on whatever sugar is already in the blood, causing your blood sugar to plunge to abnormally low levels.

Another cause of low blood sugar is exercising more than normal without adding a snack or reducing your insulin. Exercise lowers the amount of sugar in the blood. The more you exercise, the lower your blood sugar will drop. If you are taking insulin, which also lowers blood sugar, increased exercise could lead to low blood sugar.

Low blood sugar can also be caused by a successful weight-loss program. By shedding excess weight, your body's cells use insulin more effectively. In essence, your body doesn't need to produce as much insulin. If you take diabetes pills, your pancreas is being stimulated to produce insulin—perhaps more than needed for your new weight! To correct this situation, your doctor may reduce your dose of diabetes pills or eliminate it entirely.

Finally, low blood sugar can be caused by taking too much insulin. With more insulin present in the body than needed, the extra insulin works on the sugar already in the blood, resulting in abnormally low blood sugar. This is called an *insulin reaction* or *insulin shock*.

The Diabetes Control and Complications Trial showed that people who were tightly controlling their diabetes and trying to achieve normal blood sugar levels were more likely to have low blood sugar reactions. For this reason, it's very important to monitor your blood sugar more frequently and to make necessary adjustments in your treatment if you are on intensive therapy. If you do have frequent low blood sugar reactions, you may want to raise the targeted blood sugar level that you aim for to reduce the likelihood of these reactions.

If you experience low blood sugar because your insulin dose is too large, your daily dose should be adjusted. But rather than waiting three days as recommended for *high* blood sugar, a single incident of *unexplained* low blood sugar should be treated by reducing the appropriate insulin the very next day. But before adjusting insulin for low blood sugar, be sure there are no other obvious reasons for the problem. First think back and see if you can identify the reason, such as poor timing of meals, failure to eat all the food in your meal plan, exercising more than usual (without adding extra food or reducing your insulin dose), or inaccurately measuring your insulin dose.

Also, make sure that your blood sugar is indeed low. In fact, always test your blood any time you feel the symptoms of low blood sugar to be sure that's the problem. Why? Because the symptoms of other medical conditions may be similar to those of low blood sugar. If you determine that the symptoms are indeed because of low blood sugar, then follow your doctor's directions to reduce your insulin dose (if you use insulin). People who take diabetes pills and have an unexplained episode of low blood sugar should speak to their doctor about possibly reducing their medication.

WAYS TO MANAGE LOW BLOOD SUGAR

After seeking the advice of your health-care team, follow the guidelines below to treat low blood sugar.

General Guidelines

- *Treat low blood sugar immediately.* Remember, most people who use insulin occasionally experience mild insulin reactions. Some even have them frequently. Treat insulin reactions promptly, to prevent more serious problems.
- *Be prepared to treat insulin reactions at home or away.* Carry a readily available carbohydrate source such as Life Savers with you at all times (see list below). Do not eat chocolate or nuts to achieve a fast rise in your blood sugar. Such foods contain fat, which takes longer for your body to break down, and they also have more calories.
- *Don't panic.* Insulin reactions can be frightening. It's important, however, not to lose your head. Eat some carbohydrate food and allow 10 to 15 minutes for it to act. If necessary, repeat the treatment. If your next meal is not scheduled for an hour or more, have a snack such as half a turkey sandwich. If after another 10 to 15 minutes you still don't notice an improvement, call your physician.
- *Carry an ID tag.* Always carry some form of identification showing you have diabetes (see page 288).
- *Prepare for long drives.* Never drive a car for more than three hours without eating. If you experience an insulin reaction while driving, pull over to the side of the road and eat a readily available carbohydrate such as Life Savers. Wait 10 to 15 minutes before resuming your drive.
- *Adjust for weight loss.* If you are on a weight-loss program, remember that as your weight decreases, your insulin dose needs to be reduced to prevent insulin reactions. Follow the guidelines recommended by your doctor.
- *Adjust for alcohol.* Alcohol can cause low blood sugar. If you use alcoholic beverages, follow the guidelines on pages 279–282.
- *Adjust your insulin.* If you use insulin, there are several ways you can adjust for low blood sugar. They are discussed on the next few pages.
- *Monitor other medications.* Some medications can cause low blood sugar. Be sure your physician knows *all* the medications you are taking.

Carbohydrates

The following sources of carbohydrates (equal to 15 grams) are ideal for treating low blood sugar:

4 ounces of orange juice
3 ounces of regular cranberry juice
3 ounces of sweetened grape juice
4 ounces of fruit drinks such as Tang or HiC
6 ounces of regular ginger ale
5 ounces of regular soda, such as Coca-Cola or Pepsi
3–4 teaspoons of sugar dissolved in water
8 Life Savers
6 regular-sized jelly beans, or 10 small
9 small gumdrops
3 large marshmallows, or 25 small
1 tablespoon of marshmallow cream
1 tablespoon of concentrated syrup such as honey, maple
   syrup, Karo, Coke
1 small tube of cake icing (½-ounce tube)
1½ portions of dried fruits (see fruit lists on pages 319–320)
3 B-D glucose tablets
½ tube Glutose (80-gram tube)
1½ packages of Monojel

Guidelines for Adjusting Insulin

If you take insulin, there are several adjustments you may make to treat low blood sugar. For days when you are sick, please see the guidelines in Chapter 13.

- The changes you make in your insulin dose depend on the kinds of insulin you use, the time of day of injections, and the time of day the insulin reactions occur (see Table 12-1). Make your adjustments accordingly. If you use Ultralente, see the special guidelines on pages 138–140.
- If two or more of the blood tests you do each day are low, adjust first for the low test that occurs earliest in the day. Do not adjust more

TABLE 12-1. GUIDELINES FOR REDUCING INSULIN DOSES FOR LOW BLOOD SUGAR

INSULIN DOSAGE	WHEN REACTIONS OCCUR	CHANGES TO MAKE
Morning dose of NPH or Lente	Any time of day	If usual dose is less than 10 units, reduce dosage by 1 unit the next morning
		If usual dose is 10 units or more, reduce it by 2 units the next morning
Morning dose of regular and NPH or Lente	Before noon	If usual dose of regular is less than 10 units, reduce it by 1 unit the next morning
		If usual dose of regular is 10 units or more, reduce it by 2 units the next morning
	Afternoon	If usual dose of NPH or Lente is less than 10 units, reduce it by 1 unit the next morning
		If usual dose of NPH or Lente is 10 units or more, reduce it by 2 units the next morning
Dose of regular and NPH or Lente in the morning and NPH or Lente at bedtime	Before noon	If usual dose of regular is less than 10 units, reduce it by 1 unit the next morning
		If usual dose of regular is 10 units or more, reduce it by 2 units the next morning
	Noon to midnight	If usual dose of morning NPH or Lente is less than 10 units, reduce it by 1 unit the next morning

TABLE 12-1. (continued)

INSULIN DOSAGE	WHEN REACTIONS OCCUR	CHANGES TO MAKE
		If usual dose of morning NPH or Lente is 10 units or more, reduce it by 2 units the next morning
	Midnight to next morning	If usual dose of evening NPH or Lente is less than 10 units, reduce it by 1 unit the next evening
		If usual dose of evening NPH or Lente is 10 units or more, reduce it by 2 units the next evening
Dose of regular and NPH or Lente in the morning and again at dinnertime	Before noon	If usual dose of morning regular is less than 10 units, reduce it by 1 unit the next morning
		If usual dose of morning regular is 10 units or more, reduce it by 2 units the next morning
	Noon to supper	If usual dose of morning NPH or Lente is less than 10 units, reduce it by 1 unit the next morning
		If usual dose of morning NPH or Lente is 10 units or more, reduce it by 2 units the next morning
	Supper to bed-time	If usual dose of dinnertime regular is less than 10 units, reduce it by 1 unit the next day

TABLE 12-1. (continued)

INSULIN DOSAGE	WHEN REACTIONS OCCUR	CHANGES TO MAKE
		If usual dose of dinnertime regular is 10 units or more, reduce it by 2 units the next day
	During the night	If usual dose of dinnertime NPH or Lente is less than 10 units, reduce it by 1 unit the next day
		If usual dose of dinnertime NPH or Lente is 10 or more units, reduce it by 2 units the next day

than one dose or type of insulin at a time unless directed by your physician.

· If by the next day there is no improvement in your blood sugar, make the same adjustment a second time and call a member of your health-care team for advice.

Special Considerations

There are special times that you should be on the lookout for low blood sugar. These occasions are described below:

RAPID DROP IN BLOOD SUGAR. Occasionally, you may experience a rapid drop in blood sugar levels when your insulin is peaking or when you are exercising. In such situations, you may experience some of the symptoms of low blood sugar, even though your sugar level may be well above 60 mg/dl.

By testing your blood, you can determine if you were experiencing a rapid drop or actually had low blood sugar. If you feel signs of low blood sugar but are in doubt about their cause, it's best to eat some carbohydrate food rather than risk the onset of more serious symptoms.

LOW BLOOD SUGAR AT NIGHT. In adjusting insulin for high blood sugar, you should never increase your predinner or bedtime dose of intermediate-acting insulin without also testing for low blood sugar between 2 and 3 A.M. Low blood sugar that occurs at night, when you normally are asleep, is often called *nocturnal hypoglycemia*. It may be caused by too much intermediate-acting insulin in the predinner or bedtime insulin dose. Or it may result if the effect of the intermediate-acting insulin taken in the morning overlaps with the insulin taken in the evening.

You may be awakened by the low blood sugar, or you may sleep through it. When you awake in the morning, you may have a headache. Or you may remember having bad dreams or perspiring sometime during the night. Your blood sugar levels may have returned to normal. Or they may be unusually high before breakfast, due to the body's mechanism for correcting low blood sugar. This response, called *rebound*, is discussed below. By monitoring your blood sugar in the middle of the night, you can learn if your blood sugar levels are being maintained in the normal range while you are sleeping. You should perform this test anytime you increase your predinner or bedtime dose of intermediate-acting insulin.

REBOUND. Rebound, or the Somogyi effect, is caused by the body's mechanism to respond to low blood sugar. Sensing that your blood sugar levels are low, your body makes hormones that release sugar stored in the liver, raising your blood sugar level. This response—characterized by a swing from low blood sugar to high blood sugar—may take several hours to occur. This is why low blood sugar should be treated immediately with some carbohydrate.

The effects of these hormones continue even after the reaction has been treated. In fact, your blood sugar may rise to levels as high as 250–300 mg/dl or more and remain high for 12 to 24 hours, even as long as 48 hours. This condition eventually resolves itself as the extra sugar in the blood is used up by the cells or returns to the liver for storage. If you try to compensate for high blood sugar during a rebound (by taking extra insulin, eating less food, or increasing exercise), your blood sugar may swing back the other way—dropping too low after the liver has replenished its stores of sugar. Therefore during rebound, you should continue to eat and exercise as usual. You should not use extra insulin unless the high sugar levels continue for more than three days.

INSTRUCTIONS FOR CONVULSIONS OR COMA

It is unlikely that you will have a convulsion (seizure) or become unconscious during an insulin reaction. However, these serious symptoms may occur if you do not recognize the early symptoms of low blood sugar—or if you ignore them. In addition, a small percentage of people with diabetes do not experience these early symptoms and are unaware of their low blood sugar until more serious symptoms occur, such as a convulsion.

If you have a convulsion or become unconscious from low blood sugar, you should receive an injection of a hormone called *glucagon*. Glucagon is produced in the pancreas, but unlike insulin, which lowers blood sugar, glucagon raises blood sugar by stimulating the liver to release stored glucose and helping it get into the bloodstream. Glucagon should be injected into your skin (similar to the way you inject insulin) by a family member, friend, or physician, or you should be taken by ambulance to a hospital. Glucagon may cause nausea or vomiting, so you should be placed on your side when the injection is given. Under *no* circumstances should anyone try to force food or liquid into your mouth.

Once you have been given an injection of glucagon, it should take 5 to 10 minutes for the convulsions to subside or for you to regain consciousness. If your condition does not improve within that time period, you should receive a second injection.

If the convulsions do not subside or you do not regain consciousness, you should be taken immediately to an emergency room or a physician's office for treatment, which often involves injecting a glucose solution into a vein.

Once your condition has improved, eat a snack containing carbohydrate and protein, such as cola or ginger ale, followed by crackers and peanut butter or a sandwich. Otherwise, you may have another severe reaction.

Always keep glucagon on hand for an emergency. A family member or friend with whom you live should learn how to prepare and inject glucagon if the need arises. You may purchase glucagon at your local pharmacy, but you first must obtain a prescription from your doctor. Glucagon comes in a kit consisting of two items:

- a bottle of glucagon in dry-powder form
- a syringe prefilled with diluting solution.

Directions for preparing and injecting the glucagon are included with the kit. Glucagon kits are marked with an expiration date, after which their effectiveness is no longer guaranteed. Check your kit regularly to make certain the date has not expired.

SUMMARY

What to do when you experience the symptoms of low blood sugar:

1. Test your blood sugar to make sure that it's low. Compare your blood sugar with the number that your doctor gave you. If you cannot test, go to the next step.
2. If your blood sugar is low, drink or eat one of the following: 4 ounces of fruit juice, 5 ounces of regular soda, 7–8 small hard candies, or 3 glucose tablets. Be sure to carry one of these items with you at all times.
3. Rest for 10 to 15 minutes. If you still feel the side effects of low blood sugar, test your sugar level again, if possible. If your blood sugar is still low, repeat step 2. If your blood sugar continues to be low after a second dose of high-sugar food, call your health-care team.
4. If your next meal is more than an hour away, eat a snack such as low-fat cheese with crackers or half a turkey sandwich.
5. If you take insulin, adjust your dose according to the guidelines given you by your doctor.
6. If you use diabetes pills, check with your doctor to see if your medication should be reduced.
7. Figure out how your blood sugar got too low. Talk to your health-care team if it happens again.

CHAPTER 13

Treating Diabetes on Sick Days

IF YOU HAVE DIABETES, you need to take special care of your-self when you are sick. During those times, things happen in your body that will change the way it functions, including the way your cells use insulin. You must be prepared to make adjustments.

Any infectious disease, even the common cold, stomach upset, flu, or diarrhea puts stress on the human body. Stress also can result from an injury as well as surgery or invasive dental work, such as having a tooth pulled. Moreover, severe emotional trauma, such as a divorce or death in the family, also may cause bodily stress. In response to such stress, the body produces chemical messengers called *hormones*. Influenced by these hormones, the liver boosts its production of glucose. It also releases stored glucose into the bloodstream. This new supply of blood sugar provides your body with the additional energy you need to overcome an illness.

Present in large amounts, these same hormones work against the action of insulin, making the body's cells more resistant to insulin. In people who do not have diabetes, the pancreas makes up for this insulin resistance simply by increasing the secretion of insulin. In people with diabetes, the situation is vastly different. Even when you are well, your pancreas may not be able to produce enough insulin to meet your body's needs. When you get sick, the hormones described above will make your body's cells more resistant to insulin. That means blood sugar will have more trouble getting into your body's cells and will back up into the bloodstream. Also, the hormones call for the release of stored glucose, leading to a rise in blood sugar. Taken together, these responses create a potential for extremely high levels of blood sugar and a need for more insulin.

Ketoacidosis

The situation can get even more complicated. If you have Type I diabetes (insulin-dependent), the lack of enough insulin makes you unable to use the sugar in the bloodstream, and your body turns to its fat stores for energy. When this occurs, acids called ketones are produced, accumulate in the blood, and spill into the urine. The excessive formation of ketones in the blood is called *ketosis*, and the presence of ketones in the urine is called *ketonuria*.

Allowed to go untreated, the combination of high blood sugar and ketones can lead to *ketoacidosis*—an extremely serious and life-threatening condition. The condition may lead to diabetic coma and death. The symptoms of ketoacidosis are nausea, stomach pain, vomiting, chest pain, rapid shallow breathing, and difficulty staying awake.

Hyperosmolar-Nonketotic Coma

If you have Type II diabetes (non-insulin-dependent) and become sick, you should also watch out for another serious condition called *hyperosmolar-nonketotic coma*. It results from extremely high levels of blood sugar and excessive urination with the severe dehydration that can occur as a result. This problem may be caused by the stress of an illness. It can also occur in people who have had high blood sugar for a long time.

Hyperosmolar-nonketotic coma causes a severe imbalance in the body's chemistry. The body may still produce some insulin, which prevents the ketone formation seen in ketoacidosis. Nevertheless, the high blood sugar and dehydration can lead to coma or death. The symptoms that signal the onset of hyperosmolar-nonketotic coma are excessive urination, excessive thirst, increased hunger, drowsiness, nausea, vomiting, abdominal pain, and rapid shallow breathing.

Guidelines for Sick-Day Care

Ketoacidosis and hyperosmolar-nonketotic coma are very serious conditions. That's why it is extremely important that you follow the guidelines for sick-day care described below—during any period of illness or other situations associated with severe stress. By following these guidelines, you will prevent your blood sugar and ketone from rising to dangerous levels.

Treat the Underlying Illness

It's very important to treat the illness that at present has made you sick. Be sure to follow the directions of the doctor caring for your underlying illness. For example, you may be advised to use an antibiotic for an infection, or to take acetaminophen (Tylenol) or other nonaspirin medications for a fever. Always inform the doctor caring for your illness that you have diabetes.

Prevent Dehydration

When your blood sugar levels are unduly high, your kidneys cannot recycle all the sugar and the excess spills into the urine. The presence of excess sugar and salt in the urine draws additional water, causing you to pass large volumes of urine. The loss of water from your body may lead to dehydration. You can prevent dehydration by following these procedures:

- Drink one cup (8 ounces) of fluid every ½ to 1 hour. Alternate salty fluids such as broth or bouillon with low-salt liquids.
- If you are able to follow your usual meal plan, use sugar-free liquids such as water or diet soda.
- If you are unable to follow your usual meal plan (due to vomiting, etc.), alternate fluids that contain sugar (such as nondiet beverages, fruit juices, Jell-O, and Popsicles) with fluids that are sugar-free.

Prevent Hyperosmolar-Nonketotic Coma

Take the following steps to prevent this serious condition, which may occur in people with Type II diabetes:

- If you are prescribed diabetes pills or insulin, always take your medication. Never omit it, even if you are unable to eat. Check with your doctor to see if you should increase your dose during your illness.

- Monitor your blood sugar every 3–4 hours. Set your alarm clock to awaken you during the night. If you are too sick, ask someone to do the blood testing for you.
- If blood sugar levels are 240 mg/dl or higher, you should test your urine for ketones. If ketones are present, or if your blood sugar is consistently 240 mg/dl or higher, call your doctor. It's very important to watch for the presence of ketones in your urine during an illness. You can buy products to test for ketones at your pharmacy without a prescription (see Chapter 10, page 156). Your health-care team will help you choose the most appropriate product.

Prevent Ketoacidosis

This condition can lead to diabetic coma and death. To prevent ketoacidosis, it's very important to keep your blood sugar from rising too high by following these guidelines:

- Keep a bottle of regular (short-acting) insulin on hand for sick days, even though you may not normally use it. If you need extra insulin on a sick day, this will be the insulin you use. Later in this chapter are guidelines on dosage and timing of regular insulin for sick days.
- Always take your usual daily insulin dose. Never omit it, even if unable to eat, unless instructed by your physician.
- Monitor your blood sugar every 3 to 4 hours. Set your alarm clock to awaken you during the night. If you are too sick, ask someone to do the blood sugar testing for you.
- If blood sugar levels are 240 mg/dl or higher, you should also test your urine for ketones. (See page 156.)
- If ketones are present along with high blood sugar, you always need extra insulin, called a "sick-day dose." Extra insulin also is needed if blood sugar is high and ketones are not present, but you won't need as much.
- Do not use extra insulin if blood sugar is less than 240 mg/dl, even if ketones are present.

Rest and Avoid All Exercise

Do not exercise when you are sick because it can cause your blood sugar to rise. Ask someone to take care of you.

Nourish Your Body

The body needs extra energy to overcome an illness. That's why it is vital that you eat or drink some source of nourishment and calories when you are sick.

Try to eat your usual amount of carbohydrate-containing foods, including foods from the milk, vegetable, fruit, and bread/starch lists. It will help to take small amounts frequently throughout the day. Table 13-1 shows how to convert a typical meal plan into foods appropriate for a sick day. Other sick-day food suggestions appear in Table 13-2.

TABLE 13-1. CONVERTING A MEAL PLAN FOR A SICK DAY

MEAL	FOOD GROUP CHOICES	TIME*	SAMPLE MENU
Breakfast	1 milk	8 A.M.	½ cup skim milk
	1 fruit		½ cup oatmeal
	2 bread/starch	9 A.M.	1 cup tea
	1 meat	10 A.M.	4 ounces apple juice
	1 fat		6 saltines
		11 A.M.	1 cup bouillon
Lunch	2 vegetable	12 N.	1 slice toast
	1 fruit		½ cup regular Jell-O
	2 bread/starch		½ cup unsweetened canned fruit
	3 meat	1 P.M.	water
	1 fat	2 P.M.	½ Popsicle (Twin Pop)
		3 P.M.	diet ginger ale
Snack	1 bread	4 P.M.	½ cup baked custard
	1 meat	5 P.M.	1 cup broth
Dinner	2 vegetable	6 P.M.	1 slice toast
	1 fruit		⅓ cup fruit yogurt
	2 bread		diet soda
	4 meat	7 P.M.	½ cup apple juice
	1 fat	8 P.M.	1 cup tea
Snack	1 milk	9 P.M.	½ cup sherbet
	1 bread		3 saltines
	1 meat		

* To avoid dehydration, it is necessary to eat and/or drink every hour.

Table 13-2. Sick-Day Food Suggestions
(Each item equals 15 grams of carbohydrate)

apple sauce (sweetened)	½ cup	Hershey's syrup	2 tbsp
apple juice	½ cup	Life Savers	7
baked custard	½ cup	milk shake	¼ cup
Coke syrup	1½ tbsp	Popsicle (Twin-Pop)	1
cooked cereal	½ cup	pudding (sweetened)	¼ cup
creamed soups	1 cup	regular ice cream	½ cup
eggnog	½ cup	regular Jell-O	⅓ cup
fruit yogurt	⅓ cup	regular soft drinks	¾ cup (6 ounces)
frozen yogurt on a stick	1 bar	saltines	6
from container	⅓ cup	sherbet	¼ cup
grape juice	3 ounces	toast	1 slice
honey	3 tsp		

Watch for Danger Signs

Contact a member of your health-care team if you have any of the symptoms listed below. Hospital care often is necessary for these problems.

- Signs of dehydration, such as dry mouth, cracked lips, sunken eyes, weight loss, and skin that is flushed and dry.
- Inability to drink the recommended amount of fluid, or persistent vomiting for more than one hour.
- Symptoms of ketoacidosis, such as nausea, stomach pain, vomiting, chest pain, rapid shallow breathing, or difficulty staying awake.
- After taking two (2) doses of extra insulin in 24 hours, your blood sugar is still 240 mg/dl or higher.

Dosage and Timing of Extra Insulin

When you are sick, you should check your blood sugar every 4 hours. If you use insulin and your blood sugar is 240 mg/dl or higher, you should increase your dose on days you are sick. The extra amount of insulin that you need is based on the total number of units you take daily when you are well. It is usually taken as regular insulin.

Below are guidelines for increasing your insulin doses. Check with your health-care team before following these guidelines. Your doctor may recommend a different approach for your situation.

- If blood sugar levels are high and *ketones are present*, the additional insulin used as a sick-day dose of regular insulin should be 20 percent, or one fifth, of your usual daily dose. To compute the amount, divide the total number of units in your usual daily dose by 5. Take that amount in addition to your usual daily insulin.
- If *ketones are not present*, the additional insulin used as a sick-day dose of regular insulin would be 10 percent, or one tenth, of your usual dose. To compute the amount, divide the total number of units in your usual daily dose by 10. Take that amount in addition to your usual daily insulin.
- If needed, the sick-day dose of insulin should be taken following the self blood glucose testing every 3 or 4 hours for as long as the tests for blood sugar and ketones remain high. After taking two sick-day doses, call your doctor for further instructions.

Examples of Calculating a Sick-Day Dose

1. *Usual daily dose: 30 units of NPH before breakfast*

Take the following amounts of regular insulin in addition to your usual daily insulin dose:

- If blood sugar is high and ketones are present, divide 30 units by 5, which equals 6. Use 6 units of regular insulin for your additional sick-day dose.
- If blood sugar is high but no ketones are present, divide 30 units by 10, which equals 3. Use 3 units of regular insulin for your additional sick-day dose.

2. *Usual daily dose: 10 units of regular and 50 units of NPH before breakfast*

Take the following amounts of regular insulin in addition to your usual daily insulin dose:

- First compute the total number of units: 10 units + 50 units = 60 units.
- If blood sugar is high and ketones are present, divide 60 units by 5, which equals 12. Use 12 units of regular insulin for your additional sick-day dose.
- If blood sugar is high but no ketones are present, divide 60 units by

10, which equals 6 units. Use 6 units of regular insulin for your additional sick-day dose.

3. *Usual daily dose: 6 units of regular and 24 units of Lente before breakfast, plus 10 units of Lente at bedtime*

Take the following amounts of regular insulin in addition to your usual daily insulin dose:

- First compute the total number of units: 6 units + 24 units + 10 units = 40 units.
- If blood sugar is high and ketones are present, divide 40 units by 5, which equals 8. Use 8 units of regular insulin for your additional sick-day dose.
- If blood sugar is high but no ketones are present, divide 40 units by 10, which equals 4 units. Use 4 units of regular insulin for your additional sick-day dose.

Note that sick-day doses of insulin are to be taken *in addition to your usual dose of insulin*. If you test your blood and need the additional sick-day dose at a time when you normally take a dose of insulin, these extra units of regular insulin may be added to your usual dose and combined in the same syringe. If you do not know how to mix two insulins together, you can take each insulin separately.

After taking a sick-day dose, wait three to four hours and test again. If your blood sugar levels are less than 240 mg/dl, do not take extra insulin, even if ketones are still present in the urine. If blood sugar levels are still high, repeat the dose whether ketones are present or not. Test again after three or four hours. If your condition has not improved, contact a member of your health-care team. *Do not take a third sick-day dose before consulting with your nurse or doctor*. Sometimes people who are sick hesitate to use extra amounts of insulin. If you are not sure how much extra insulin to take, contact your physician.

In addition, people who are not normally on insulin may be put on insulin temporarily to keep their blood sugar under control when sick, or if they will be undergoing surgery or have a serious injury. Often, once the surgery or illness has passed, they will be taken off insulin.

Part Five

SPECIAL CHALLENGES OF DIABETES

CHAPTER 14

Diabetes in Children

IF YOUR CHILD HAS diabetes, you probably have plenty of questions at the tip of your tongue: *What should I do when my child's blood sugar is too high or too low? What can my child eat? How do I take care of my child on a day-to-day basis? How will I find a reliable baby-sitter? What should I do if my child has the flu?*

Before answering these and other questions, it's important to emphasize that medical experts know much more than ever about treating diabetes in children. There are many forms of insulin that can help you keep your child's blood sugar under acceptable control. You have access to glucose monitors to help you, and your child's other caregivers, monitor your child's blood sugar. And your health-care team is available to provide the education and support you and your family need.

The key is to approach your child's diabetes in an organized and positive manner. Children have an amazing capacity to adapt. In fact, they often are more able than adults to accept changes in their lifestyle, primarily because they have not yet developed habits that are hard to break. With your help—coupled with the expert advice from a health-care team—your child can continue to lead a happy, healthy, and active life.

BASIC SKILLS FOR CAREGIVERS

When your child is diagnosed with diabetes, your first step as parents or caregivers is to focus on the immediate treatment program that your child needs. In time, you can learn more about the intricacies of diabetes—knowledge that will make you even more aware of the various treatment options and better able to help your child live well. But you should learn about diabetes gradually. It's unrealistic to try to learn everything at once. You'll just become confused and overwhelmed. This is not the time to worry about the possible problems that may occur in people who have had poorly controlled diabetes for a long time. There will be plenty of time to develop strategies that will help prevent these long-term complications. Start by learning to cope with the basics!

What Parents and Caregivers Need to Know

As your child's caregiver, your first goal is to learn the following "survival skills":

- *insulin injections*—how to fill a syringe and give insulin injections
- *low blood sugar*—how to recognize, treat, and prevent low blood sugar
- *high blood sugar*—how to recognize, treat, and prevent high blood sugar
- *monitoring*—how to monitor your child's blood sugar and urine ketone levels
- *nutrition*—what kinds of food to prepare, how much to offer, and when to offer these foods
- *exercise*—how to adjust insulin and food intake for times when your child is physically active
- *rules for sick days*—how to handle your child's diabetes during sick days

In this chapter, you will become acquainted with these skills. For more detailed information, be sure to read the other chapters on these topics. And, of course, continue to rely on your child's health-care team as your primary source of information. They will tell you what you need to know for your child's diabetes. In this chapter, you will learn the ways diabetes can affect normal behavior at various stages of your child's development. Understanding these changes is a very important part of your child's care.

What Your Child Needs to Know

How much does your child need to know about his or her diabetes? It all depends on your child's age and maturity. Some children can learn to measure and inject their own insulin by the time they are about 12 years old. However, it is recommended that parents and caregivers share responsibility with their children for insulin injections until puberty is completed, usually by mid-adolescence. Every child is different in his or her capacity to cope with the demands of diabetes, but all children need and deserve their parents' help and support well into the teenage years. Before you give your child the responsibility for measuring and injecting insulin, remember that this is a serious and complex matter. Your child needs to be mature enough to handle the job, and in general, children are not capable of having sole responsibility for insulin injections until they are 15 years old.

How about monitoring? Children need to understand the rationale for regular blood sugar monitoring, whether or not they can do these tests themselves. Most important, they need to learn the symptoms of a "low blood sugar reaction" (also called an insulin reaction) and take the appropriate action. Later, as they begin to appreciate the overall goals of their diabetes treatment, they will want to accept a greater role in their care. In fact, children quickly learn that maintaining good health is the ticket to joining their friends in many of the normal activities of youth.

A Message to Parents: Handle Your Emotions

As you learn about the basic skills of caring for your child, it's important to focus on your thoughts and feelings. First, think about how you initially reacted to the news that your child has diabetes. Perhaps you felt overwhelmed, confused, or angry that this happened to your child and your family. You may even have felt guilty because you mistakenly blamed your child for being lazy or cranky, when, in fact, diabetes was causing most of the problem. These feelings are all part of the normal "coping" process that begins at diagnosis.

If you can eliminate such negative feelings, you'll be less likely to fall into an emotional trap that can stand in the way of managing your child's diabetes. Below are some positive attitudes to develop in caring for your child.

Learn to Share Responsibility

As a parent, you will be carrying most of the burden for caring for your child's diabetes. In essence, you are the one who will help plan, carry out, and assess your child's treatment.

You should expect a change in your family's dynamics. In raising any child, a parent's goal is to gradually transfer responsibility to that child. But when a child has diabetes, it's not quite the same. You will have to achieve a more delicate balance between encouraging your child's independence and still requiring a level of dependence. It is very important to talk with your health-care team about this very significant parenting issue.

Sometimes, you may believe *you alone* can meet your child's special needs. But you should realize that it's necessary to transfer some responsibility to other people—family members, relatives, school staff, coaches, and friends. They, too, can learn what the symptoms of low blood sugar are and how to treat this problem. Your health-care team can be an important resource in helping you to educate family, school personnel, and friends about diabetes.

Present a United Front

At first, parents often feel fearful and frustrated about their child's diabetes. In that frustration, they may blame each other's family for "causing" the diabetes, perhaps blurting out, "It didn't come from our side of the family!" As parents, you should not waste valuable emotional energy on this issue. The fact is that no one really knows how your child developed diabetes. It's far better to rally around a common goal, presenting a united front to help your child!

Be Positive, Honest, and Hopeful

If your child has diabetes, the whole family needs to be involved. At times, this may cause a strain on the family's ability to understand and support your child and you. Sometimes you will feel very alone. Perhaps your child is the only person you know who has diabetes, particularly if you live in a small town. In the United States, about 100,000 children and teenagers have diabetes. This means only 1 of every 700 people develop diabetes before age 19. If you feel alone in the struggle, you may become despondent and fail to do some of the things you should be doing to help your child. As parents you may be going through other struggles such as financial pressures or trouble at work, which may also get in the way of your child's treatment, perhaps causing you to give up and essentially leave your child "on his own."

How can you cope? Be honest about all your feelings. First of all, talk them out with your child's health-care team. They can help you face the situation realistically—and with a great deal of hope. They can help you keep your child's welfare in the forefront. Secondly, connect with other parents of youngsters with diabetes. Ask your health-care team to help you meet others in a similar situation, or contact the American Diabetes Association or Juvenile Diabetes Foundation for information on family support groups in your area.

Remember, children often take their cues from their parents. If you maintain a "can do" spirit, it will rub off on your child. You will also be able to teach your child more about diabetes. For example, your child may think that diabetes will just disappear someday. Diabetes, however, will never go away. It will be with your child *forever*, and you need to help your child accept this fact.

WHY DO CHILDREN DEVELOP DIABETES?

Children develop diabetes for the same reasons that older people do. In the case of Type I diabetes—the commonest form of diabetes in children—hereditary factors may have set the stage. In other words, your child may have been born with certain genes, the basic blueprints of life, that increased the chance of developing diabetes. Then something comes along that triggers the immune system to mistakenly destroy the body's own cells—the beta cells in the pancreas that produce insulin. Once this happens, the child has diabetes. Perhaps that "something" is a viral infection. Or perhaps the normal stress on the body from the rapid growth of puberty causes the immune system to destroy the beta cells.

Most children develop Type I diabetes, also known as "insulin-dependent diabetes" because they must depend on insulin injections to live. In fact, this type was often known as "juvenile diabetes" until scientists discovered that Type I diabetes can occur at any age. It affects both boys and girls in equal numbers.

In children, the symptoms of Type I diabetes usually evolve rapidly. This is in sharp contrast to adults, who may develop Type I diabetes more slowly. In children, the symptoms include tremendous thirst and frequent urination. They also may have a recurrence of bed-wetting. The child may continue to have a good appetite and eat large amounts of food, yet experience an unexplained loss of weight. If the condition is not recognized early, dehydration may occur due to the loss of water from excessive urination. Vision can be blurred from temporary changes in the lens of the eye. Overall, an active and robust child becomes weak, irritable, and has little energy. Schoolwork often takes a plunge. The child may also complain of pains in the legs and abdomen or have difficulty breathing.

When the onset is abrupt, a proper diagnosis can be made quickly. At times, however, the symptoms of diabetes may be confusing to a parent, as they may resemble a "flu" or stomach virus or a urinary tract infection. However, a physician who is familiar with these symptoms should give the child a blood test, and if the test shows an elevated blood sugar level, diabetes will be diagnosed. When sugar levels are high in the blood, there usually is sugar in the urine as well as ketones.

Children may also develop a rare form of Type II diabetes (non-insulin-dependent), referred to as "maturity-onset diabetes of youth." These children usually are very overweight teenagers. A special test may be necessary to diagnose this type of diabetes.

STAGES OF DIABETES IN CHILDREN

Children often go through the following stages of diabetes:

- *Acute onset* or *newly diagnosed*—This is the first sign that your child has diabetes. Symptoms include fatigue, frequent urination, thirst, and, of course, high blood sugar. During this stage, your child's blood sugar levels may be controlled with small doses of intermediate-acting insulin, with or without regular insulin, once or twice a day.
- *Remission* or *"honeymoon"*—During this stage, your child's diabetes seems to improve or even go away. This "remission" usually lasts only a short time. The diabetes has not been cured. Soon, it will come back and become even a greater challenge to control. During this stage, it's important to continue your child's insulin doses, even if only one or two units are given each day. (There is growing evidence that even tiny doses of injected insulin may be protecting the remaining beta cells, and it may be possible to prolong the honeymoon stage this way.) The remission often ends with an infection or another acute illness, or with the onset of puberty and increased growth.
- *Intensification*—During this stage, managing your child's diabetes becomes more intense. Diabetes is not getting worse, but it is more difficult to control. You must closely monitor your child's blood

sugar levels, and the amount or types of injected insulin may have to be increased or adjusted. You and your child may get discouraged because the blood sugar levels tend to fluctuate so much without any obvious cause and despite your careful efforts.

· *Total diabetes*—At this stage, the pancreas's beta cells have been totally destroyed. The body depends solely on an outside supply of insulin to convert food into energy or store it for future use. Diabetes becomes somewhat harder to control because the body is no longer producing any insulin to supplement the injected insulin. If insulin injections are omitted, your child is at immediate risk of developing *ketoacidosis*, a dangerous condition caused by the buildup of ketones in the blood (see page 165).

THE TREATMENT PLAN

In managing diabetes in children, one goal of the treatment plan developed by your health-care team will be to relieve the symptoms caused by your child's high blood sugar levels. It will also work to prevent severe acute complications such as ketoacidosis and diabetic coma. Moreover, the treatment plan will reduce your child's chances of developing long-term complications from diabetes. As your child follows this plan, he or she will feel better and have more energy.

Blood sugar levels have an impact on how your child grows and develops. For this reason, your child's blood sugar levels should be as well-controlled as possible. While this may seem difficult at times, it should be your overall goal. But always approach the treatment plan with a bit of realism. It is important that children feel included in family, school, and holiday celebrations, and there may be times that to maintain the social and emotional health of your child, you have to compromise. For example, it is unrealistic to try to "fine tune" blood sugar levels at a child's birthday party.

Your Health-Care Team Is Vital

If your child has diabetes, it's vital that you seek the guidance of a health-care team. The team should consist of people with a special knowledge and interest in how children develop—both physically and emotionally. They should also have up-to-date training and experience in the management of Type I diabetes.

The team should include a pediatrician who is specially trained in diabetes, a pediatric diabetes nurse specialist, a mental-health professional (a social worker or a clinical psychologist who understands emotional and social problems in the family), and a dietitian who works mostly with children and teenagers to help them understand nutrition and meal planning. The team should work with the child's own pediatrician and others involved with the child, such as teachers, the school nurse, school guidance counselor, and sports coach.

Your health-care team is there for you now and in the future. At first, it will help you and your child understand and follow the initial treatment plan. The team will also help you continue the treatment into the years ahead, making the proper adjustments as your child grows and develops. This support is an important part of the overall treatment.

If you don't live near a medical center that is staffed with a diabetes treatment team, your child will probably receive routine care and emergency treatment from your local doctor. But you may find it very beneficial to travel occasionally to a center that has a specialized diabetes department. If you choose this course, it's essential for everyone concerned—you, your family doctor, and the members of the child's treatment team—to maintain constant communication.

Insulin

Insulin is the primary treatment for young people with diabetes. Before your child developed diabetes, insulin was present at all times in the bloodstream. The pancreas automatically secreted insulin in response to eating, and the level of insulin increased with the amount and nutritional content of food eaten. Now that your child has diabetes and is being treated with insulin injections, the goal is to try to copy that pattern as closely as possible. In general, one daily injection usually won't be enough. Most children with Type I diabetes need several daily injections. And they usually need two types of insulin—short-acting and intermediate-acting—to keep blood sugar at the desired level. The insulin dosing programs outlined in Chapter 8 for Type I diabetes may be also used in the treatment of children and teenagers; please study this chapter to gain an understanding of various dosing schedules.

Some people with diabetes use a treatment program called "intensive diabetes therapy." In this program, which is described in Chapter 9, insulin doses are changed daily, based on the results of frequent testing of blood sugar. It is usually not recommended for young children, who are not yet able to recognize the symptoms of low blood sugar and participate in their treatment plan.

Your child's insulin therapy probably will be adjusted during the four stages of diabetes described above. During the "acute onset" stage, the treatment will vary depending on the blood sugar levels. These levels are fairly stable, so doses usually change only with variations in food consumption and activity. In this stage, children usually require one or two injections of one or two types of insulin. In the remission stage, your child's diabetes may be managed with small doses of intermediate-acting insulin. Even though diabetes may seem to have "disappeared," always continue to give some insulin.

Once the intensification stage or total diabetes is reached, your child will need to follow a "mixed-dose" insulin program. That's when two types of insulin are mixed in the same syringe. The dose is often "split"—given more than one time during the day. Children usually require two or three injections of insulin during these stages of diabetes.

The following program is often effective for children, but always check with your health-care team before using any dosing schedule:

- a morning mixed dose of short-acting and intermediate-acting insulins
- a second injection before dinner using either a mixed dose of short-acting and intermediate-acting insulins or a dose of short-acting insulin and a third injection at bedtime of intermediate-acting insulin

The purpose of the dinner or bedtime intermediate-acting insulin is to minimize high sugar levels at night, which might be indicated by nighttime urinating or bed-wetting or by very high blood sugar before breakfast.

How much insulin does your child need? Your doctor will determine the precise amount to use, depending on your child's needs. These needs are likely to change as your child develops, so it's important that your child be reevaluated at least every three months or at time intervals recommended by your health-care team.

Exercise can reduce the body's insulin needs, although it will *never* totally replace injected insulin (see Chapter 5). If your child's activity level varies, it may be necessary to adjust his or her insulin dose. For example, if your child is going away to summer camp or starting an active summer job after an inactive school year, he or she may need less insulin, more food, or both.

How do you determine when an adjustment is necessary? Any adjustments to your child's dose will be based on the results of blood sugar tests taken over a period of time, three days or perhaps longer. If a definite pattern is observed, your health-care team will advise you to make a change in the insulin dose. Changes should not be made more often than once in three days, unless a severe high or low sugar occurs or you are instructed to do so by your health-care team.

When should you give the injection? It should be given 30 *minutes before meals*, unless your child's blood sugar is less than 70 mg/dl. This allows the short-acting insulin to be in the bloodstream, ready to begin working when the food is eaten. If your child eats immediately after the injection, his or her blood sugar levels will rise much faster.

Both parents and all your child's daily caregivers should learn to prepare and give insulin injections. Detailed guidelines are provided in Chapter 8. At about age 12, children may begin to give their own injections, but only with strict parental guidance. Don't rush your child to accept this responsibility until he or she is mature enough to understand the dangers of injecting an inaccurate dose of insulin.

Nutrition

The nutritional needs of children with diabetes are the same as those of children who don't have it. Your child needs no special foods, vitamins, or minerals. The eating program that your dietitian will develop provides everything needed for energy and growth. However, the key to meal planning is to coordinate eating with the action of insulin and with your child's exercise. This topic is discussed in detail in Chapter 3.

Your child should try to eat meals and snacks at about the same times daily according to the meal plan. The total number of calories as well as the proportions of carbohydrate, protein, and fat should be consistent from day to day. However, your child's eating program should be reviewed at least once a year, due to changes in each child's growth patterns and need for calories. As a general rule, a child of average weight at age 1 needs about 1,000 calories daily, with 100 calories per day added for each year up to the onset of puberty (age 11–14). For example, the daily needs of a 10-year-old would be 1,000 plus 1,000 (100 × 10), for a total of 2,000 calories daily. There are exceptions to every rule, however, and each child's needs must be considered on an individual basis.

It's important to coordinate eating with insulin's time of action.

Whenever insulin is at its peak, there should be enough sugar in the blood for it to act upon. If not, your child's blood sugar may drop too low. To minimize the likelihood of having low blood sugar, your child will need snacks between meals and at bedtime. Most teenagers can eliminate the midmorning snack, but even so, they should always have some carbohydrate on hand, just in case their blood sugar drops too low (see list of foods on page 172).

Many youngsters are influenced by peer pressure about food—pressure to eat something, not to eat something, or to lose weight. The fear or embarrassment of having a low blood sugar reaction in front of their friends may cause teenagers to overeat. Children sometimes test the limits of their diabetes by experimenting with overeating and undereating. In striving for independence, they may try to manipulate their parents by eating improperly. In dealing with these issues, the approach should be similar to the way families can effectively solve other types of parent-child conflicts. Try to get to the bottom of the issues causing the conflicts. Set firm, but realistic guidelines in consultation with the dietitian on their health-care team.

Exercise

Exercise is a good way to lower blood sugar levels, along with the use of insulin and a meal plan. In fact, a program of regular exercise actually allows young people with diabetes more food choices.

LOWERING BLOOD SUGAR. The benefits of exercise for diabetes are discussed in Chapter 5. In summary, exercise will lower blood sugar at the time the exercise is done. Low blood sugar can also occur after exercise, a "lag" effect caused by the body's cells becoming more sensitive to insulin. This effect persists even when the person has stopped exercising. In addition, once exercise is completed, the body works to replenish the storage form of glucose (glycogen), drawing upon sugar in the blood. As a result, the blood sugar levels may drop even farther. Additional food is usually needed to prevent these drops in blood sugar.

There are times when your child's overall activity will increase, such as during summer vacations. At those times, your child may need less insulin. Your doctor will help you determine the dose.

Teenagers may be taught to reduce their insulin dose when they participate in sports. The amount of the reduction depends on the results of blood sugar tests done before and after exercise. Parents and teenagers should check with the health-care team about making such adjustments to the insulin dose.

BEWARE OF HIGH BLOOD SUGAR. There are times that exercise can actually cause blood sugar to *rise* and can lead to the production of ketones. This can happen with vigorous exercise done by someone with poorly controlled Type I diabetes. If your child has high blood sugar of 240 or more and ketones in the urine (or 400 mg/dl or higher without ketones), he or she should not do any strenuous activity until the situation is brought under control. For more information, see the discussion in Chapter 5.

MONITORING DIABETES IN CHILDREN

Testing Blood Sugar

Home testing of blood sugar, also called monitoring, is a good way to watch your child's daily blood sugar patterns. It allows you to make decisions about how to manage any variation in your child's lifestyle. The concept and techniques behind monitoring are covered in detail in Chapter 10 and also in Chapter 13, where you'll find special guidelines to follow when your child is sick.

At times, you may think of monitoring as a bothersome chore, something forced upon you and your child by your health-care team. Instead, see monitoring for its many benefits. It is a very effective tool to evaluate how well your child's diabetes is being managed. Such checks will help you determine if your child's blood sugar is too low or too high. The test results will also give you an idea of how to make adjustments in food and insulin to match your child's activity level.

Most children tolerate blood testing well. Many school-age children are able to use glucose monitors and perform the test by themselves. There is no right age to learn—only the right time for that child. But you and your child don't need to become slaves to the task. The best approach is knowing how and when to monitor and what to do with the results. Monitor only as necessary. Repeated testing is a waste of time and money unless the results are used to help adjust insulin, diet, and exercise to improve control of your child's diabetes.

Ask your health-care team for times that you should monitor your child's blood sugar. They will tailor a monitoring program specifically to your child's needs. Diabetes experts recommend that children have their blood tested at least two times a day. Twice a week, you should plan to perform four tests during the day—before the three main meals and before the bedtime snack. And each month, perform two blood glucose tests at 2 to 3 A.M. to see if your child's blood sugar is in control during the night. A blood sugar test should be performed at bedtime if there has been increased physical activity during the day. Any bedtime blood sugar less than 120 mg/dl may require an increased amount of bedtime snack.

Whenever you monitor, write down test results and show this record to your health-care team. Be sure to note any significant variations in activity or food consumption. Using this record, your health-care team can spot patterns in your child's blood sugar levels and make appropriate adjustments.

When checking blood sugar, try to avoid using the words "test" and "good" or "bad" to describe the results. A child or teen may think you are being judgmental, which can cause resentment and anger, feelings that may lead them to lose interest in controlling the diabetes. Children have been known to give false results in order to please their parents. The words "high" and "low" are more appropriate to describe blood sugar levels.

Glycosylated Hemoglobin

This test, described in Chapter 10, is also called hemoglobin A_1 or A_{1C}. It provides a good idea of how well your child's blood sugar has been managed over the past 2 to 3 months. This test is particularly useful with children because their blood sugar levels fluctuate, making it hard to assess the results of regular blood tests. But remember, the results of the glycosylated hemoglobin test represent only an average of what the blood sugar levels have been. Therefore, the test should never be used as a substitute for blood sugar testing. It should only be used in addition to daily monitoring.

Your health-care team may set a goal for your child's A_{1C} levels. At the Joslin Diabetes Center, the normal A_{1C} range for people without diabetes is 4.0 to 6.0 percent. For adults with diabetes, "excellent control" is an A_{1C} level under 7 percent. However, the activity level and eating habits of children vary, so reaching a level under 8 percent can be difficult or unsafe. Keep in mind that goals must be tailored to each child, and, as discussed earlier, the test your doctor's lab runs may have a different "normal" range.

DIABETES AND CHILD DEVELOPMENT

The treatment of children with diabetes will vary according to their stage of growth and development. As a parent, you should be aware of the different forms of treatment required at different ages.

Infants and Very Young Children

Increasingly, diabetes is being found in children under age 5. Infants need relatively small amounts of insulin, so you or your pharmacist probably will be advised to dilute the clear (regular) insulin from the usual U-100 strength to U-50 (half strength), to U-25 (quarter strength), or to U-10 (tenth strength). To make these dilutions, use the diluting solution provided by insulin manufacturers. Your doctor or nurse educator can tell you how to make a proper mixture with as low a dilution as you need. Be aware that the amounts of insulin needed will increase as your child grows.

Through Age 12

Many youngsters can master some parts of their diabetes care. Before age 12, they can be actively involved in meal planning, learn to spot symptoms of low blood sugar and how to treat it, and help with blood testing. But your child probably won't be ready to take responsibility for injecting insulin until after age 12, so you shouldn't hurry the child into taking on this responsibility. It's critical that insulin be given at the right time and at the right dose. If not, serious results can occur.

Once children reach a maturity level that allows them to take on more of their diabetes treatment, parents should continue to oversee all aspects of care. Some parents are overly concerned that unless their child takes full responsibility early on, the child will end up being too dependent as a young adult. This is not true. Your child will eventually learn to accept his or her role in self-care. Older children are often eager to take over the injections when there are personal payoffs, such as an overnight visit to a friend's house or going on a camping trip or class outing!

What about your child's growth? Before physicians understood the effects of chronic high blood sugar on growth, some children with diabetes didn't grow to normal heights. That picture has completely changed! Today, with modern insulin and monitoring methods, children treated with usual insulin therapy (two to three daily injections) who achieve reasonably good control of their metabolism will grow at a normal rate. If your child's growth and development are not proceeding as expected, check with your doctor. You may need to pay closer attention to diabetes control, or your child may need a change in treatment plan. Of course, there are other reasons for poor growth and development unrelated to diabetes. Your doctor can help find and treat these problems.

Teenagers

All children—whether they have diabetes or not—gradually learn to accept responsibility and strive for independence. When a child has diabetes, this quest for independence is more complicated. All children in their teens undergo rapid growth and sexual changes. For a child with diabetes, these bodily changes make it harder to control blood sugar. The upshot is that teenagers with diabetes need closer medical supervision—just when they want to be more independent and "do their own thing." They may also be at a stage where they temporarily reject the values of their parents or other authority figures. Diabetes often becomes the battleground for this struggle. Some teens test the limits of their condition, wanting to find out whether they *really* have diabetes and what happens if they don't follow their treatment program. This may mean overeating, omitting insulin injections, or refusing to do blood testing.

The teen with diabetes is quite sensitive to "being different." He or she may omit insulin injections, eat spontaneously with his or her peer group, and omit monitoring in order to prove "nothing is wrong." As a parent, you should expect such lapses once in a while, tolerating them up to a point. However, if your teen shows severe self-destructive behavior—actions that result in repeated episodes of ketoacidosis and numerous visits to the emergency room—it is a signal that the family needs the help and support of a professional counselor. In such cases, your nurse educator, psychiatric social worker, or clinical psychologist can be very important members of your teen's diabetes treatment team.

Puberty and Menstruation

In general, the onset of puberty usually proceeds on schedule in children with diabetes. Poor diabetes control, however, can delay puberty. For example, in girls it may mean a delay in menstruation, which can cause great anxiety and distress for the child and her parents. But be assured that if the thyroid function and other hormones are normal, this delay corrects itself as your daughter's diabetes control improves. During menstruation, many women notice a rise in blood sugar levels for a few days just before the beginning of the monthly flow. At these times, your daughter may need to temporarily increase her insulin dose. Boys don't experience such dramatic changes.

EVERYDAY ACTIVITIES

School

Children with diabetes can participate fully in all school activities. But they should understand the need to keep their diabetes well regulated during the school day. This will not only help them in their normal growth and development, but also help minimize high or low blood sugar reactions that may be distressing and call attention to them as "different."

Teachers should be told about your child's diabetes, but must not shelter or overprotect the youngster by making obvious allowances, for example, letting your child do less schoolwork than classmates. Parents should meet with the child's teacher at the beginning of every year to explain the nature of diabetes and describe the need for snacks and for eating meals on time. Most important, your child's teacher should be informed about low blood sugar reactions—how to recognize and treat them. School nurses and other school staff may also be part of your child's care away from home. It is useful to prepare written instructions for your child's teachers.

Organized Sports

Youngsters with diabetes are encouraged to participate in athletic activities of all types. Just be sure that your child's coaches and teammates know about the possibility of a low blood sugar reaction, what the symptoms are and how to treat this problem. On the days of strenuous activity, your child may need to monitor blood sugar and eat more. He or she should also keep some carbohydrate on hand to deal with low blood sugar. Diabetes is not an obstacle to success in sports. There have been several professional athletes—in baseball, hockey, and other sports—who have effectively managed Type I diabetes.

Leaving the Child with a Baby-sitter

It's important for parents to get away, even if it's just for an evening out, but finding a baby-sitter may be a little more difficult. Set aside time to teach the sitter the basics of diabetes care and what to do in emergencies (a quick review is provided in Chapter 23). Make sure the sitter knows how to recognize and treat low blood sugar. If you are to be away for more than an evening, invite the person to come a day or two earlier while you are home to learn your child's normal day-to-day routine for handling diabetes.

A phone call can solve many problems. Always leave the phone number of the family doctor and the phone number and address where you can be reached. Many parents carry a beeper so they can be reached easily.

Camps and Other Special Programs

Just because your child has diabetes doesn't mean he or she must be excluded from summer camp. Since the 1920s, camps have been available for young people with diabetes. Your child might benefit physically and emotionally from one of these camps, as well as learn more about diabetes.

There are regular camps with staff who can care for children with diabetes. There are also camps devoted just to children with diabetes. Joslin Diabetes Center runs the Elliott P. Joslin Camp for Boys in Charlton, Massachusetts, and provides medical staff for the Clara Barton Camp for Girls, in nearby Oxford, Massachusetts. For lists of camps in the United States, contact the American Diabetes Association (see resource list in Chapter 24). There are also camps in other countries.

The primary purpose of these camps is to provide fun and recreation while also ensuring good diabetes treatment and helping children learn more about managing their disease. A successful camp experience often leaves children feeling less isolated and more comfortable with themselves. They can gain confidence in caring for their diabetes and also see how their peers cope with similar situations. Camp also relieves the anxiety and depression that some children feel for being "different." An added bonus is that such camps also provide parents with several care-free weeks away from the day-to-day care of their child. Everyone gets a vacation!

CHAPTER 15

Diabetes and Pregnancy

THANKS TO IMPROVEMENTS in diabetes management over the past 50 years, women with diabetes can now give birth to healthy babies. In fact, infant survival rates for women with diabetes are now nearly identical with those for nondiabetic women.

Today, women can control their diabetes by monitoring their blood sugar at home and making adjustments in their insulin doses. In addition, there are numerous medical tests to monitor the well-being of the mother and child throughout the months of pregnancy. Such medical advances have significantly reduced the risks of pregnancy to the mother and improved the chances of survival for the unborn baby. However, it's important to realize that diabetes *does* make pregnancy more difficult. And babies born to diabetic women do have an increased risk of birth defects. But if good diabetes control is achieved before conception, the risks of miscarriage and also the risk of birth defects in the baby are greatly reduced.

Before you get pregnant, your doctor should perform certain tests to see if your diabetes is controlled well enough to support carrying a baby. This "good control" must continue throughout the pregnancy. It requires a strong commitment from a mother who is willing to check her blood sugar four times a day and review the results with her diabetes doctor on a weekly basis. In addition, women with diabetes usually need to be in the care of an obstetrician who deals with "high-risk" cases. And after delivery, the baby may need the care of a doctor who specializes in the care of newborns.

How Is Pregnancy Different If You Have Diabetes?

All pregnant women, whether they have diabetes or not, require more insulin than they did before they got pregnant. This is because the placenta, which provides nutritional support to the growing baby, produces hormones that make insulin less effective. As the placenta grows, more insulin is needed to keep blood sugar normal. By the end of pregnancy, women generally need up to twice the amount of insulin that they did before becoming pregnant.

The shortage of insulin can create problems with the type of nutritional fuel the body burns during pregnancy. In general, the body gets its energy from blood sugar (glucose). If there isn't enough insulin in the bloodstream to help convert the available sugar into usable energy, the body turns to fat and protein for energy. In *any* woman who is pregnant, the body is more likely to turn to fat than protein, saving the protein for the growth of the baby.

Women who don't have diabetes generally can keep up with the increased need for insulin during pregnancy. They continue to use blood sugar efficiently. But pregnant women with diabetes—who don't have enough insulin to meet their needs—are more likely to burn fat instead of sugar. When this happens, blood sugar and ketones can build up in the bloodstream, leading to the dangerous condition called *ketoacidosis* (see page 165). Preventing this condition is one of the main reasons that you must take special care of yourself during pregnancy. You must regularly monitor your blood sugar and test your urine for ketones.

Preexisting Diabetes

If you had diabetes and needed to take insulin *before* you became pregnant, then you probably will need to take more during the time you carry your baby. In fact, by the time you are close to delivery, you will need much more—often twice as much. In addition, your diet must contain more calories, including more carbohydrate and protein to provide for your needs and those of your developing child. During your pregnancy, you will have to pay special attention to the balance of insulin, food, and physical activity. With the advice of your health-care team, you probably will need to make many adjustments to your treatment program.

Gestational Diabetes

Above-normal blood sugar can develop in women who did not have diabetes before they got pregnant. Why does their blood sugar rise? Because the pancreas, which under normal circumstances is able to supply enough insulin, can't keep up with the increasing demand for insulin during pregnancy. This condition is called *gestational diabetes* because gestation refers to the time that the baby is developing in the womb. This form of diabetes is more likely to occur in women who are overweight or over age 30, also those who have a family history of diabetes. However, gestational diabetes may occur in women who have no known risk factors for this condition.

Most women who have diabetes during pregnancy find out during the course of the pregnancy itself, often as a result of routine testing done by their doctor when they are 24 to 28 weeks pregnant. First a *glucose loading test* is done, in which the blood sugar is checked 1 hour after drinking a sugary drink. If the blood sugar is high at this time, the obstetrician will recommend a *glucose tolerance test* (discussed in Chapter 1), which measures the blood sugar for 3 hours after a sugary drink.

The most important act in treating gestational diabetes is maintaining a proper diet. Insulin is only rarely needed to keep blood sugar in control. And even if a woman does have to take insulin, she usually does not need insulin injections after the baby is born. But she should keep in mind that she may develop diabetes later. Some women with gestational diabetes need to continue taking insulin after delivery. In such cases, it is likely that they were in early stages of diabetes anyway, and the pregnancy just made it obvious.

If you ever have had gestational diabetes, be sure to tell any future doctors you may consult during a subsequent pregnancy—or for any reason—so they can keep a lookout for changes in your metabolism. To decrease the risk of developing diabetes in the future, you should do regular aerobic exercise (see Chapter 5) and try to maintain your weight as close to normal as possible.

PLANNING PREGNANCY

The decision to become pregnant is very personal. If you have diabetes and are considering having a baby, the best way to ensure your baby's healthy development is to be sure that you have excellent control of your diabetes *before* you become pregnant. Your doctor will review your blood sugar test results with you and help you adjust your insulin dose until your blood sugar goals are achieved. Your doctor may also recommend that you start taking prenatal vitamins before you become pregnant. Recent studies have demonstrated that one of these vitamins, folic acid, reduces the risk of certain birth defects.

Many women wonder if pregnancy will worsen any complications they already may be having from diabetes. To answer that question, your doctor will do a full evaluation. It is advisable to have such an evaluation *before* getting pregnant. That way, your health-care team can inform you of any additional risks that you may face during your pregnancy. While some complications of diabetes may temporarily worsen during pregnancy, after the baby is born a woman usually returns to the level she might have expected if she hadn't been pregnant. However, you and your health-care team should pay special attention to the following conditions that can be dangerous, even if they worsen just for a short time:

Retinopathy

One of these serious conditions is a change in the blood vessels on the retina, the delicate, light-sensitive membranes lining the back of the eye. Called *retinopathy*, this condition is discussed in detail in Chapter 17. If you have this problem and it has reached the stage in which new, undesired blood vessels are forming on the retina (*neovascularization*), you may lose your vision. Getting pregnant can make matters worse, because pregnancy can speed up the changes in the eyes associated with diabetes. If new blood vessels are detected, you should postpone your pregnancy.

Another eye problem, called "background retinopathy," often occurs in people with diabetes. With this condition, the risk of losing sight is much lower than with the condition described above. Background retinopathy may progress somewhat during pregnancy, but it usually doesn't get to a threatening stage.

If you have diabetes it is very important to know the condition of your eyes, especially if you are considering pregnancy. Your eyes should be evaluated by a physician called an *ophthalmologist*, particularly one who is an expert in diagnosing and treating diseases of the retina. If retinopathy is detected and it is in a risky stage, your doctor may advise you to postpone pregnancy to avoid more severe damage. Retinopathy can be successfully treated with laser therapy, and once stabilized, it is much less likely to get worse during pregnancy.

All pregnant women with diabetes should get their eyes checked by an ophthalmologist two or three times during pregnancy. If the condition of the eyes worsens, the doctor will be able to detect the problem early on and begin treatment without delay. As with other complications from diabetes, any eye changes you have during pregnancy may improve gradually after delivery.

Kidneys

Before you become pregnant, it also is a good idea to check how well your kidneys are functioning. Your doctor can determine this by performing simple tests on your urine. If your kidneys are functioning well, they will very likely continue to do so during pregnancy. If, however, protein is being lost in the urine, pregnancy can make the problem worse. It can lead to high blood pressure (*hypertension*) and your body may begin to retain fluids (*edema*). Once this occurs, you must take great caution and care. You even may need prolonged bed rest at home or in a hospital. Sometimes premature delivery of the baby is necessary to protect the health of the mother.

Neuropathy

Even with good diabetes control, damage to your nerves (*neuropathy*) can get worse during pregnancy. The symptoms include tingling, numbness, or discomfort in the leg or foot. See Chapter 17 for more information on relieving the symptoms of nerve problems.

Managing Diabetes During Pregnancy

If you have diabetes and are pregnant, it's best if you are cared for by a team of experts in this area of medicine. Such a team is made up of a diabetes specialist (*endocrinologist*), an obstetrician who specializes in high-risk pregnancies (*perinatologist*), an eye specialist (*ophthalmologist*), a nurse educator, a dietitian, and a psychological counselor. Another person who should be present at the baby's delivery is a specialist in the care of newborn infants (*neonatologist*).

If you don't live near a diabetes care center where such a team would be available, consult your primary doctor as well as your obstetrician and pediatrician. Overall, you will need two kinds of care—for your diabetes and for your pregnancy—and this care should be closely co-ordinated by all members of your health-care team.

THE COURSE OF PREGNANCY

First Trimester

As soon as pregnancy is diagnosed, you should begin visiting your health-care team on a weekly basis. The first trimester (the first three months) is critical to the developing child (fetus). During this time, the basic body structures begin to form, and if diabetes is uncontrolled, there could be major structural damage to the fetus, resulting in birth defects.

At your first visit, you should see your diabetes specialist and your obstetrician. In addition, it is important to see a nurse educator, who will review the goals of home care during pregnancy, and a nutritionist, who will prescribe a revised diet that includes additional calories to cover the increased needs of your pregnancy. Iron and vitamin supplements are usually prescribed. Close and frequent monitoring of your blood pressure, weight, and eyes is important. If your pregnancy causes nausea and vomiting—called "morning sickness," even though it can occur at any time—your insulin doses may be decreased a little at first.

Throughout your care, urine cultures are frequently done to make sure you don't have a urinary tract infection. Such infections can affect diabetes control and must be treated. If you develop a fever, cloudy or bloody urine, urinary burning or urgency (constantly feeling that you have to urinate), contact your doctor at once. In the later stages of pregnancy, it is sometimes difficult to tell the symptoms of urinary infection from the pressure of the baby on the bladder, so let your doctor decide what is actually happening.

Second Trimester

During the second trimester (months 4 to 6), weekly checkups should continue. Also, you will continue closely monitoring and caring for your diabetes. For many women, their diabetes at this time becomes more stable than in the first trimester, although the insulin dose may have to be increased. During this period, your health-care team will watch closely for increases in blood pressure, fluid retention, and decreases in kidney function. In addition, various tests may be done to determine the health of the developing baby. Anemia is also a common problem during this period, and treatment with iron supplements may be necessary.

Third Trimester

Weekly checkups continue through the third trimester (months 7 to 9). For many women, their diabetes remains relatively stable, although the insulin dose may have to be increased. Many women need twice as much. Also, the mixture of insulins may have to be changed. As with all diabetes, insulin adjustments vary from person to person. Your goal is good control, regardless of the insulin dose that is needed. Often, toward the last few weeks of pregnancy, the amount of insulin needed will begin to decline.

During the third trimester, any signs of high blood pressure, fluid buildup, or kidney problems are of concern. An ultrasound test (described later in this chapter) is performed periodically to check the baby's development, and the baby's heart is closely monitored. Additional tests may be performed, some of which are routinely done for all pregnancies—for example, testing the hemoglobin level in your blood to make sure you are not anemic. Other tests may be done, based on your specific situation. For example, your doctor may want to measure your thyroid function.

MONITORING THE MOTHER'S HEALTH

Throughout your pregnancy, the goal of your diabetes treatment program is to achieve blood sugar levels as close to normal as possible. Of course, this level may vary from person to person. Ideally the goal is a blood sugar level of 60 to 100 mg/dl before breakfast (fasting level) and 100 to 140 mg/dl one to two hours after eating. To achieve this control, you should test your blood at least four times a day: before breakfast and two hours after breakfast, lunch, and dinner. Before adjusting your insulin doses, consider all other possible reasons for any change in your blood sugar levels—what you ate, the timing of the insulin dose in relation to meals, or any changes in your physical activity.

Adjusting Your Meal Plan

The expression "Now you're eating for two!" takes on added meaning for pregnant women who have diabetes. As with your regular diabetes care, your diet is a very significant part of your treatment during pregnancy.

For this reason, you should meet early on with a dietitian skilled in nutrition for pregnant women with diabetes. Together, you will develop a meal plan for the first trimester of pregnancy. At the beginning of the second trimester, this plan may be changed to meet the increasing needs of the growing baby. Your meal plan will be based on the general principles discussed in Chapter 3. However, during pregnancy, you will need extra calories and will also probably be advised to take supplements of vitamins and minerals, such as iron, folic acid, and calcium. In addition, you may need more between-meal snacks because in all pregnant women, the metabolic needs increase.

Adjusting Insulin

Guidelines for adjusting insulin doses are found in Chapter 8. In general, you can use the same insulin types you used before your pregnancy. Three or four daily injections are usually needed to achieve near-normal blood sugar levels. This is called "intensive diabetes therapy" and is discussed in Chapter 9. Research has shown that precise control during pregnancy is important to the health of the fetus.

During pregnancy the body's cells become more resistant to insulin. As a result, the blood sugar rises more rapidly after eating, reaching a higher peak, and then drops more rapidly to lower levels before the next meal. To respond to this pattern, you should wait 30 minutes after taking your insulin before you eat your meal to allow some insulin to be in your bloodstream to react with the sugar from the food you will eat. You may need a greater amount of short-acting insulin (regular) and less intermediate- or long-acting insulin in the mixed dose of insulin taken before meals. You may also need to eat more snacks between meals to help prevent low blood sugar that may occur before the next meal.

Treatment involving an insulin pump may be needed for women who are unable to achieve good control with multiple injections. As with all other methods of insulin treatment, good blood sugar control using an insulin pump should be established before pregnancy.

The benefit to the fetus of near-normal blood sugar should be balanced with the risk to the mother of having a severe low-blood-sugar reaction. People who no longer can tell when their blood sugar is low are particularly at risk (see Chapter 12). If you have a low-blood-sugar reaction, you may lose control of your car while driving, lose consciousness, or have a seizure. You may be unable to take anything by mouth to raise your blood sugar into the normal range. In these infrequent situations, an injection of glucagon can be given (see pages 177–178). Family members should be taught how to give such an injection.

Testing for Ketones

Your doctor also will ask you to test your urine for ketones, due to the increased risk of ketoacidosis during pregnancy (the test for ketones is described on page 156). Ketoacidosis can be dangerous to both you and your baby. You should check for ketones each morning before eating or before taking insulin. If ketones are present for two days in a row, even though your blood sugar is normal or close to normal, you should call a member of your health-care team. The causes vary, but you may need a larger nighttime snack.

On days when you are feeling well and your blood sugar is above 240 mg/dl, always check for ketones. Call your doctor immediately if ketones are more than a "trace." On days when you are sick, it's even more important to monitor for ketones—even if the illness is minor, such as common cold, upset stomach, flu, or diarrhea. (To learn how to take care of your diabetes on sick days, see the guidelines in Chapter 13.) Why is all this monitoring so important? Because you need to do everything you can to prevent ketoacidosis, which can harm both you and your baby, and could ultimately lead to the death of the fetus. Fortunately, since the advent of home blood sugar monitoring and intensive management, ketoacidosis is quite rare.

Good control of blood sugar also can help prevent *preeclampsia*, a condition that is defined by a combination of findings—high blood pressure, protein in the urine, and fluid retention. It is more likely to occur in young women and those with preexisting high blood pressure and a previous pregnancy complicated by preeclampsia. Preeclampsia can progress to a serious condition called *eclampsia*, which involves seizures. (This problem is different from the impairment of kidney function described earlier in this chapter.) Preeclampsia can occur in people who do not have diabetes. But the problem is more common in people who have diabetes. By closely monitoring your health, your doctor will be able to diagnose preeclampsia early and begin treatment. This often includes bed rest at home or hospitalization. If preeclampsia is severe, the baby may have to be delivered early to protect the health of the mother. This could have ill effects on the baby, since the baby's lungs may not be able to support life on their own. A respirator may be necessary to help the baby breathe. Occasionally, very premature babies may die.

MONITORING THE BABY'S HEALTH

Depending on your specific needs, your health-care team may decide to perform a variety of tests to make sure that your baby is developing properly. These tests will also help predict the time of delivery.

- *Alpha-fetoprotein*—This is a blood test that is performed at 16 to 18 weeks to detect possible defects in the brain or spinal cord of the baby. Since the test is not very precise, an ultrasound is performed if it is abnormal to further evaluate the fetus.
- *Ultrasound*—This test uses sound waves, which pass through the mother and fetus and are translated into images of your baby's internal organs and bony structures. This test does not use x-rays, which may be harmful to a developing fetus. Ultrasound is usually first performed at week 16 or 18 and is used to estimate the expected delivery date. It is usually repeated between weeks 26 and 28, and again near the time of delivery to be sure that the baby is growing properly and to measure weight and size. The size is important in determining whether the baby can be delivered normally or if a cesarean delivery (surgery) will be necessary. Additional ultrasound tests can and may be done, e.g., to assist in performing the amniocentesis.
- *Nonstress test*—This test uses a sound pickup device, but it is different from the one used for ultrasound. Often done in the last few weeks of pregnancy, it measures the heart rate of the baby as it changes with movement.
- *Oxytocin challenge test* or *stress test*—In this test, also done in the final weeks, a small amount of medication is given to the mother to cause a small uterine contraction. The response of the baby's heart is then observed.
- *Amniocentesis*—This test on the fluid surrounding the baby is used to check the baby's lungs. A needle is passed through the skin (after it is numbed) and uterus into the fluid. Higher "test scores" mean the baby's lungs are more mature and less likely to have trouble

breathing at birth. Amniocentesis can also detect a range of birth defects including genetic abnormalities.

Proper nutrition is very important to the health of you and your baby. If you have any of the problems found in the list in Table 15-1, call your doctor or dietitian.

TABLE 15-1. WHEN TO CONTACT YOUR DIETITIAN DURING PREGNANCY

You should contact your dietitian (or physician) for a review of your eating program if you notice any of the following:

1. KETONES are present in your urine when your blood glucose level is within or near the normal range. This may indicate you are not eating enough food and particularly that you need a large evening snack.
2. WEIGHT LOSS. This may indicate that you are not eating enough food.
3. INADEQUATE WEIGHT GAIN (less than 2 pounds per month during the second and third trimester). This may indicate that you are not eating enough food.
4. EXCESSIVE WEIGHT GAIN (more than 1 pound per month in the first trimester and thereafter 7 pounds or more per month or more than 2 pounds per week). This may indicate that you are eating too much food or that your body is retaining fluid.
5. WIDELY FLUCTUATING BLOOD GLUCOSE LEVELS. This may indicate that you are eating too much food during certain times of the day. (You should be sure to contact your physician for this problem in particular.)

WEIGHT GAIN AND EXERCISE

Weight Gain

Your meal plan will be designed to help you gain weight during your pregnancy. This weight gain is important to ensure the proper growth of your baby. In addition, you need to have enough carbohydrate in your diet so that your body doesn't burn fat for energy, leading to the production of ketones. How much weight should you gain? First, check the weight chart on page 88. If you are currently at about the correct weight for your height, you should plan to gain about 24 to 28 pounds during pregnancy. If you are overweight, you should gain only 15 to 24 pounds. If you are underweight, you may gain 28 to 32 pounds.

About half of the weight gained during pregnancy is due to the growth of tissues in the mother that support the growth of the fetus (extra blood, breast enlargement, and fat stores). The other half of the weight gain is for the baby itself, the *placenta* (the tissue in the womb that supplies nourishment to the baby), and the *amniotic fluid* (the fluid that surrounds the fetus).

Your health-care team will closely monitor your weight during pregnancy. How fast weight is gained will vary from woman to woman. But on average, expect to gain only about 3–5 pounds in the first trimester. Then during the second and third trimesters, expect to gain about ½ to 1 pound per week. Try to gain weight gradually. If you are losing weight, your health-care team will want to evaluate and treat the problem.

Physical Activity

If you have diabetes and are pregnant, you may continue to do forms of exercise that are mild and safe. In fact, most women with diabetes can continue the exercise plan they had prior to becoming pregnant. But this is not a time to start a new and involved program of physical activity. As with all women who are pregnant, you must be careful as your pregnancy progresses. The extra weight you are carrying in your abdomen causes a change in your center of gravity. And rather than engaging in activities that can more easily throw you off balance, choose forms of exercise that are safer, such as walking on a well-paved sidewalk or in a shopping mall.

DELIVERY

Women with diabetes are no longer routinely hospitalized before delivery. One day beforehand, an amniocentesis is performed to document that the baby's lungs are mature. Delivery is usually scheduled at 38 weeks. But some women with uncomplicated pregnancies whose diabetes has been in excellent control may be safely delivered at 39 to 40 weeks (full term). And once the baby is born, he or she is often cared for in the newborn intensive care unit of the hospital, where he or she can be closely observed.

Based on the estimated size of the baby and the presence or absence of serious retinopathy, your doctor will recommend either a delivery through the birth canal (vaginal delivery) or a cesarean delivery (surgery). If a vaginal delivery is planned, you will receive an intravenous solution containing Pitocin, a synthetic hormone that stimulates the uterus to contract. On the day of your delivery, you will receive only a fraction of your usual morning dose of insulin.

As soon as the baby is born, the mother's need for insulin drops significantly. For a few days, in fact, you may need less than what you used before pregnancy. However, as your body returns to normal, your insulin needs will probably be about the same as before you were pregnant.

BREAST-FEEDING

Breast-feeding is encouraged for women with diabetes. However, you may prefer to bottle-feed your baby. The decision will depend on personal choice and the advice of your doctors.

If your baby needs to be in a newborn intensive care unit, that will present an obstacle to breast-feeding. To deal with this situation, during the first three days after delivery, most babies are given bottles of formula to keep their blood sugar from dropping too low. You should request breast pumps to stimulate nursing until your milk comes in, usually three days after delivery. At this time, you will be able to adequately nourish your infant.

Women who breast-feed often need an increase in diet, similar to what they ate while pregnant, but this varies from person to person. You may be advised to eat a snack before nursing to prevent low blood sugar. Also, be sure to get enough calcium in your diet. If you notice any inflammation or soreness in your breast (often due to infection), contact your doctor, who can help determine the cause and best plan of action.

YOUR DECISION

The decision to become pregnant requires more thought and planning if you have diabetes. But it's comforting to know that medical science has reduced your risks so significantly. Today, many women with diabetes are successfully giving birth to healthy babies. The decision is ultimately yours to make. But always talk it over with the prospective father and your doctor. Together, you can decide on what's best for you and your family.

CHAPTER 16

Diabetes and Sexual Issues

A PERSON DIAGNOSED WITH diabetes often asks, "Will diabetes or its treatment affect my sex life?" After all, people with diabetes have the same sexual desires as everyone else. The good news is that, in general, people with diabetes are able to perform sexual activities normally and lead satisfying sex lives. However, in both men and women with diabetes, some problems related to sexual function can occur.

SEXUAL FUNCTION IN MEN

Impotence

One problem with sexual function that any man can develop—whether he has diabetes or not—is impotence, the loss of the ability to achieve or maintain an erection of the penis sufficient for sexual function. It can be a very frustrating problem. In the general population, the leading causes of impotence are psychological—things that happen in the mind. The problem can be brought on by tension, fear of failure, guilt, or other such factors. Men with diabetes also are subject to these tensions, so psychological factors must be considered as the possible cause of their impotence. In such cases the impotence is not directly related to diabetes.

Physical factors can also play a role in causing impotence. Some of these factors are directly related to diabetes; others are of a more general nature. Impotence caused by the physical effects of diabetes usually occurs after a man has had diabetes for a number of years, particularly if his diabetes has been poorly controlled. Some experts believe that the main cause is *neuropathy*—that is, damage to the nerves that control an erection. Nerve damage can result from chronically high levels of blood sugar, which explains why men with poorly controlled blood sugar are at higher risk for impotence.

The nerves involved in an erection work by controlling small valves that are located in the blood vessels leading to and from the penis. Sexual stimulus opens the valves that control the inflow of blood, permitting it to fill spongy areas within the penis. The outflow valves do just the opposite; they close, trapping the blood within the penis and keeping it erect. When the sexual stimulus subsides, the process reverses; the blood drains out, and the penis becomes flaccid. When impotence occurs in men with diabetes, it may be due to damage of the nerve fibers that control these valves. As a result, the valves don't function properly. But keep in mind that nerve damage from diabetes can occur in other parts of the body as well, a topic discussed in Chapter 17.

In other men (with or without diabetes), the cause of impotence may be the hardening of blood vessels that supply the flow of blood to the penis. These blood vessels become narrowed or blocked, similar to vascular disease that occurs in other parts of the body.

Whatever the cause, the development of impotence in men with diabetes tends to come on gradually; it doesn't suddenly occur one evening. Over time, the man will notice that his penis is less rigid or that he can't maintain an erection for as long a period of time. Nighttime and morning erections are also affected. With this decline, the man doesn't necessarily feel a loss of sexual desire. That's why impotence can be so frustrating. However, it does not mean that the man is infertile. He simply is unable to perform sexually.

One of the problems in discussing impotence is that no one really knows what is "normal." Modern life tends to emphasize sex—in the news media, advertising, literature, and movies—which raises people's expectations to unrealistic levels. However, we do know that impotence can occur at any age, and the result is sometimes the opposite of what we might expect. For example, some men who have diabetes can perform sexually into their seventies, while some men who do not have diabetes experience impotence in their forties or fifties. And some men who become impotent due to diabetes are not as disturbed as they thought they would be. In general, these men have built a solid basis for their emotional life, with many other interests and with a happy marriage. They realize that the impotence is not their fault and is nothing to feel guilty about. It's simply a physical fact of life.

Men with diabetes who are experiencing impotence should first discuss the problem with their doctor. Sometimes it can be caused by medications used for other medical conditions. Your doctor can also test to see if the production of your sex hormones is normal. In addition, you may be advised to be evaluated by a *urologist*, a doctor who specializes in the urinary tract, as well as a psychologist, who can help you sort out any stresses in your life.

Various treatments for impotence have been developed. The most effective involve a penile *prosthesis*. Such devices are surgically inserted into the penis by a urologist. There are two basic types of prostheses. One model is permanently elongated and can be bent down when not in use, but the length and rigid nature will remain. The second is an inflatable type. A small pump, placed under one of the testicles, is used to pump balloonlike cylinders full of a fluid that is stored in a reservoir in the lower groin. When this model is not in use, the penis appears normal in size. Using either model, men who are otherwise fertile may be able to ejaculate semen normally. In general, both types have been widely and successfully used.

There are other treatments for impotence that do not require surgery. Vacuum devices are one such approach. With this method, a cylinder is placed over the penis and held tightly against the body. A tube at the end of the cylinder leads to a pump that draws air out of the cylinder, which creates a vacuum that pulls blood into the penis to cause an erection. A special elastic device is then slipped around the base of the penis to hold in the blood during sexual activity (maximum time is about one-half hour). Removing the elastic allows the blood to flow out and the penis to become smaller again. Injection therapy is another option. With this approach, substances are injected into the penis that cause blood vessels to contract, leading to the trapping of blood and a temporary erection.

If you are experiencing impotence, a member of your health-care team can discuss the various treatments available and determine what is best for you.

Retrograde Ejaculation

Another problem that a small number of men with diabetes face is known as *retrograde ejaculation*, which refers to a backward flow of semen, the fluid that contains sperm. Normally, during sexual activity, the semen is ejaculated outward. But some men with diabetes have a type of nerve damage that allows the semen to flow backward into the bladder, where it is destroyed. If this occurs, fertility can be reduced or prevented altogether, a serious problem to young men wishing to start a family.

The nerve damage that causes retrograde ejaculation is different from the damage that results in impotence. And fortunately, the condition is quite rare. Ask your physician if you have any early signs of this problem. Such signs may be an incentive for you and your partner to begin having children sooner, rather than later. But remember, there are many other causes of infertility. If a couple is experiencing any difficulty in conceiving a child, both partners should be checked by a fertility expert.

SEXUAL FUNCTION IN WOMEN

Women with diabetes should also be aware of bodily changes that can have an effect on female function and sexuality. A major decision in the life of a woman is whether or not to become pregnant. If she has diabetes, it is especially important that her diabetes is under excellent control *just before* and *during* pregnancy. For more information on this topic, see the discussion in Chapter 15.

Menstruation

Another area related to female function is menstruation, the regular monthly flow of blood from the uterus. Some women with diabetes notice a rise in blood sugar levels for a few days just before the monthly flow begins. If you notice this pattern with menstruation, your health-care team may advise you to increase your insulin at this time. Poor control of diabetes (with chronically high blood sugar) may cause a delay in the onset of puberty or may create menstrual irregularities.

Vaginal Dryness and Infections

Some women with diabetes notice that the vagina doesn't naturally become lubricated with sexual activity. This can make sexual relations uncomfortable, and while the problem can occur in all women, it may be more likely in women with poorly controlled diabetes. Also, high levels of blood glucose may make women more susceptible to vaginal yeast infections, which, in turn, can make intercourse more painful. If you are having vaginal problems, talk to your doctor or nurse educator. They may be able to recommend medications or lubricants that will increase your comfort. And renew your efforts to get your diabetes in control.

ISSUES FOR BOTH MEN AND WOMEN

Urinary Tract Infections

People with diabetes, particularly those with poor control, are more prone to urinary tract infections. This is because in the presence of high blood sugar, the cells of the immune system are less effective in destroying bacteria that enter the body. Urinary tract infections can make sexual activity very uncomfortable, especially in women. If you have cloudy or bloody urine, burning in the urinary tract, or constantly feel as if you have to urinate, contact your doctor immediately. The infection should be treated at once with antibiotics before it has a chance to spread to your kidneys. Do not have any sexual relations until it is cleared up.

Genital Infections

Compared with the general population, people with poorly controlled diabetes tend to have more problems with genital infections caused by types of fungus commonly called "yeast." These infections, which can be very annoying, affect the vagina or the tip of the penis and are usually related to poor diabetes control, which reduces the body's ability to resist infection and also leads to high sugar content in the urine, which encourages the growth of these organisms. The condition can be treated with medicated creams and ointments. Check with your doctor about which product is best for your particular infection. However, keep in mind that these organisms are often resistant to any treatment until your diabetes control is improved. So get back on track as soon as possible.

Similar to the general population, people with diabetes can contract sexually transmitted infections. People with diabetes who are sexually active should have regular medical examinations to screen for such problems.

Birth Control Options

Because it is vital that women with diabetes have their blood sugar under control *before* becoming pregnant, birth control measures for women with diabetes become more important as a means of preventing pregnancy until all conditions are optimal for mother and a developing fetus.

In general, women and men with diabetes use the same birth control measures as people who don't have diabetes. Among them are *oral contraceptives* ("the pill"), which have been used by millions of women for the past few decades. The birth control pills of the 1970s had much higher doses of hormones (estrogen and progestin) than those used today. Women with diabetes who choose oral contraceptives should choose a low-dose "combination" pill of estrogen and progestin or a "mini" pill containing only progestin. In most cases, insulin needs do not change on low-dose pills, but women with diabetes should have their blood pressure, glycosylated hemoglobin, cholesterol level, and eyes checked regularly—before and during the use of oral contraceptives. If used properly, oral contraceptives are highly effective in preventing pregnancy. But they do not protect against sexually transmitted diseases, so condoms are recommended for additional protection.

The use of a *diaphragm*, a flexible device placed in the woman's vagina to block the passage of semen, is another way of preventing pregnancy. This method is still widely used. *Intrauterine devices* (IUDs) can be used by some women with diabetes. But due to the risk of pelvic inflammation from IUDs, this method is generally reserved for women who have completed their childbearing, are in a monogamous relationship, and have no history of pelvic inflammatory disease. *Condoms* are thin latex sheaths that cover the penis and are used in combination with spermicide creams in preventing pregnancy. They also reduce the risk of contracting the AIDS virus and other sexually transmitted diseases from sexual partners.

At some time in your life, you or your partner may want to consider more permanent ways to prevent pregnancy. In men, this may be done through *vasectomy*, in which part of the sperm-carrying duct is removed. Women may wish to consider *tubal ligation*, in which the fallopian tubes from the ovaries to the uterus are tied off. Although these procedures are usually permanent, they will not impair sexual function or enjoyment. Clearly, there is no single form of contraception that is perfect for everyone. Your doctor will help you and your partner decide what's best for your situation.

Sexual Activity and Low Blood Sugar

Some people with diabetes are concerned that the exertion of sexual activity may cause them to have a low-blood-sugar reaction, similar to what can happen with other forms of physical activity. As with exercise, however, the situation varies from person to person. If you experience low blood sugar after sexual activity, correct for it the same way as with other types of exercise—by adjusting your insulin or eating a snack (see Chapter 5). For example, you might try drinking a sugar-containing beverage just before sexual relations or possibly eating a snack afterward. Monitoring your blood sugar before and after sex can help determine the timing and amount of the snack.

PREMARITAL COUNSELING

If you have diabetes, the prospect of marriage often raises several issues. For example, you may wonder, "Will my children have diabetes?" The answer to that question is very complicated and, as noted earlier, the percentage of risk depends on which type of diabetes you have, whether one partner has diabetes or both of you do, or who in your extended family has the condition. Your doctor can help you sort out answers to this important question.

You may also wish to consider a few other issues. A lifelong condition such as diabetes can pose certain problems in a marriage, which, in turn, require a lot of patience and understanding by everyone in the family. If you have diabetes and are thinking of getting married, you should talk it out honestly with your prospective spouse. Once you both understand all the potential problems that may arise, you will be better able to handle them. Below are a few topics you may wish to address:

- At present, there is no "cure" for diabetes. People with diabetes can and do lead active and productive lives. But it requires a *lifelong commitment* to medical care. That's why it's important for prospective partners of people with diabetes to understand the basics about diabetes and its care. They should also be prepared to support their spouse's self-care program.
- *Complications from diabetes*, such as problems with the eyes, kidneys, and nerves, may occur after a number of years (see Chapter 17). You and your prospective partner should be aware of these problems and the effects they may have on your marriage.

- *Pregnancy* in a woman with diabetes may be more difficult and require more attention than in women who don't have diabetes (see Chapter 15). However, in recent years, medicine has made great strides in this area, and risks of complications have been greatly reduced.
- Special problems with *employment* and *insurance* may arise, issues that must be handled with understanding, planning, and sensitivity.

Of course, all couples must deal with the ups and downs that life together can bring. In the marriage of a person with diabetes, knowledge and understanding by both partners, aided and abetted by generous doses of love, can go a long way toward creating and sustaining a stable and happy relationship.

CHAPTER 17

Long-Term Complications of Diabetes

IF YOU HAVE EITHER Type I or Type II diabetes, you should be aware that your diabetes can cause a number of problems that develop after you've had the disease for many years. These long-term complications can appear in various parts of your body—your eyes, kidneys, nerves, blood vessels, and other areas—and they are more likely to occur if your diabetes has not been well controlled. That's why it's so important to work with your health-care team to develop a program that keeps your blood sugar as close to normal as possible to minimize or prevent these complications.

The landmark research study called the Diabetes Control and Complications Trial (DCCT) has shown that people with Type I diabetes can reduce their risk of developing complications by 50 percent or more by keeping excellent blood sugar control, i.e., maintaining blood sugar levels as close to normal as possible throughout the day. To gain this type of control, you may want to consider using "intensive diabetes therapy," which involves testing your blood frequently throughout the day and, based on the results, adjusting your insulin doses. This approach is discussed in Chapter 9.

Researchers at Joslin Diabetes Center believe that people with Type II diabetes can also benefit from intensifying their diabetes treatment to achieve as close to normal blood sugar as is safely possible. For example, if you currently are trying to control your diabetes with diet and exercise, do the best possible job in following your meal and exercise plan and test your blood sugar daily to see how your efforts are working.

If your control is not as good as possible using that strategy, your doctor may add diabetes pills to your treatment program. Or if you are currently using diabetes pills, your doctor may start you on insulin. The message is clear: Whether you have Type I or Type II diabetes, you should work with your health-care team to achieve blood sugar levels as close to normal as possible to reduce your risks of long-term complications.

Some people discover that, despite their best efforts, their diabetes is so difficult to manage that they can't achieve the type of control they want. Despite their hard work, some people still develop complications. This can be very discouraging. But remember, by doing the best job you can with your diabetes day-to-day, you *are* lowering your risks of developing further complications later on, and are slowing the progress of complications that may be just beginning.

THE EYES

Your eyes are very vulnerable to the effect of diabetes. For example, many people have *blurred vision* in the early stages of diabetes. It is the result of fluid seeping into the lens of the eye, causing it to swell and altering its ability to focus properly. Once diabetes treatment begins, the lens resumes its normal shape and vision improves. Blurred vision can also result from fluctuating blood sugar. In such cases, the damage is not permanent. It lasts only a few weeks until you get your blood sugar in control.

You also may have other eye problems, many of which are not related to diabetes. For example, anyone can get *glaucoma*, which is caused by too much pressure in the eye. In fact, everyone past age 40 is at risk for all types of glaucoma. People with diabetes, however, have a greater risk of developing glaucoma. Your eye doctor can diagnose glaucoma with a simple test that measures your eyeball pressure. If detected, glaucoma should be treated promptly with, for example, eye drops that cause proper fluid exchange.

Another problem that anyone can develop is *cataracts*, a condition in which the lens of the eye becomes cloudy. This problem usually comes with advancing age, and everyone is at risk. People with diabetes, however, are more likely to develop cataracts at a younger age. Poor diabetes control can speed up the process of developing cataracts. Eye doctors can treat cataracts with surgery.

All of the above conditions can occur in anyone, whether the person has diabetes or not. But there are some serious eye problems that are directly related to poorly controlled diabetes.

Retinopathy

The most serious eye problem that can occur with diabetes is damage to the *retina*, the thin, light-sensitive inner lining in the back of your eye. This damage, called *retinopathy*, occurs to small blood vessels in the retina which are easily harmed by high levels of glucose in the blood. About 90 percent of people who have had diabetes more than 25 years will have some blood vessel changes in their eyes. Fortunately, complete blindness is rare if retinopathy is diagnosed early and treated promptly and correctly. As a matter of fact, many people who have blood vessel changes in their eyes don't realize it until their doctor tells them. So yearly eye exams by an ophthalmologist are a must for people with diabetes. Also, there are many advances in treating and preventing eye disease associated with diabetes. We truly have entered a new era of hope that serious eye damage can be treated and prevented.

How does retinopathy occur? To understand the problem, you first need to know how the eye works. The eye looks like a Ping-Pong ball and functions like a camera, with a lens in front and other structures in back (see Figure 17-1). For you to see, light bounces off an object and then passes through your eye's lens, which focuses it on your retina. The retina translates the light signal into nerve impulses, which travel to the optic nerve at the back of your eye. The optic nerve then sends

Figure 17-1

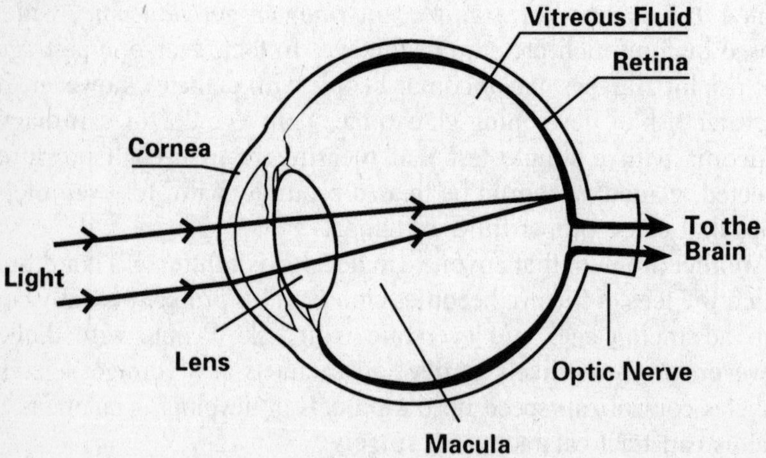

the message to your brain, which interprets the image. Wherever there is damage to the retina, the eye is unable to send these messages to the brain.

There are two stages in diabetic retinopathy—an initial stage, which may be called nonproliferative retinopathy, and a more serious stage called proliferative retinopathy, in which there is a greater loss of vision or even total blindness (see Figure 17-2). Another condition, called diabetic macular edema, can occur with either stage.

In the early nonproliferative stage (called also *background retinopathy*) high levels of blood sugar cause damage to the blood vessels in the retina. They actually can leak fluid, which can collect and cause the retina to swell. When fluid collects in the central part of the retina (*macula*), it may swell (*macular edema*), resulting in blurred vision. Macular edema can be treated with laser surgery when central vision is threatened.

A more dangerous stage of eye disease from diabetes is *proliferative retinopathy*. During this stage, abnormal blood vessels grow over the surface of the retina. These fragile blood vessels may rupture and bleed into the *vitreous humor*, the clear gel that fills the center of the eye. When this happens, the blood blocks the passage of light to the retina and loss of vision or even blindness may occur. A further problem can occur when these blood vessels cause scar tissue, which may pull on the retina and cause it to become detached from the back of the eye. This type of retinopathy can also be treated with laser surgery to reduce the risk of vision loss. If hemorrhage does occur and vision is lost, vitrectomy surgery (a process to remove the blood from within the eye) can frequently successfully restore vision.

Figure 17-2

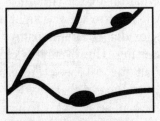 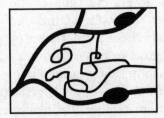

Background or early
diabetic retinopathy
(nonproliferative)

Proliferative or
advanced diabetic
retinopathy

Preventing Eye Disease

To reduce your risk of all forms of retinopathy, you should maintain your blood sugar levels as close to normal as possible. You should also have your eyes examined at least once a year, and perhaps more frequently. Your doctor will refer you to an *ophthalmologist*, a specialist in eye disease. You should also check your blood pressure frequently because high blood pressure increases your risk of retinopathy.

If you experience any changes in your vision, notify your doctor immediately. An eye examination can determine the cause of your vision change, and you can begin timely treatment. Today, treatment can dramatically reduce your risk of severe visual loss. Techniques include *laser surgery*, in which a bright powerful beam of light is focused on the retina. The light "burns" the area of the retina affected by retinopathy, stopping the formation of new blood vessels. Laser surgery is usually done on an outpatient basis in the eye doctor's office. It may cause some minor discomfort, but that disappears quickly. After treatment, you may experience a slight decrease in vision. But the overall benefits far outweigh any minor drawbacks. The technique is a virtual eyesight-saver.

Remember, your eyes can become damaged without your knowing it. The damage can occur in areas that do not affect vision. And you often feel no pain. Only careful eye examinations at regular intervals will detect the damage. If you have Type I diabetes (insulin-dependent), it's a good idea to have your eyes examined by an ophthalmologist at least once a year. If you have Type II diabetes (non-insulin-dependent), your eyes should be examined by an ophthalmologist when your diabetes is diagnosed and at least once a year afterward. Under certain circumstances, you may need immediate attention. Call your eye doctor's office if you experience any of the following symptoms: sudden loss of vision, severe eye pain, or the sensation that a curtain is coming down over your eyes. Your doctor will want to see you right away.

Presently there is no known cure for diabetic retinopathy, and no known means to prevent it from occurring. However, it is clear from major, nationwide clinical studies that the risk of severe vision loss (being able to see only the largest letter on the eye chart five feet in front of you) from proliferative retinopathy can be reduced to less than 5 percent, and the risk of moderate vision loss (your vision decreasing by 50 percent) from diabetic macular edema can be substantially reduced by proper eye care and laser treatment when necessary.

What can you do to preserve your vision? While there is no foolproof system to prevent retinopathy, whether you have Type I or Type II diabetes, the most important things are:

- Maintain as good control as possible of your blood sugar levels, blood pressure, and blood cholesterol levels.
- Have at least annual, complete eye examinations through dilated pupils by an eye doctor experienced in diagnosing and managing diabetic eye disease.
- Remember that appropriate laser treatment and surgery can significantly reduce the risk of vision loss and blindness from diabetes.

You are a key player in preventing eye complications related to diabetes. Research shows that you may be able to reduce your chances of eye damage by maintaining good control of your blood sugar. To do that, you need to see your health-care team at least twice a year (and ophthalmologist yearly), monitor your blood sugar, take your medication, follow a meal plan, and exercise regularly. Your sight is so important. You'll want to do everything possible to keep it!

Figure 17-3

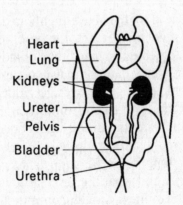

Heart
Lung
Kidneys
Ureter
Pelvis
Bladder
Urethra

THE KIDNEYS

Your kidneys also are at risk of damage from high blood sugar. The most serious kidney disease is called *nephropathy*, which can occur in people who have had diabetes for a long time, particularly diabetes that is poorly controlled.

Kidney damage is a serious problem, because your kidneys are very important organs. Each person is born with two kidneys, which lie toward the back of your body, one on either side of the spine and slightly above the waist (see Figure 17-3). As blood flows through the kidneys, tiny filtering units called *nephrons* filter out waste products and other substances, passing them out as urine. Over a period of time, high blood sugar can damage these filtering units, making it impossible for them to carry out their job. Once the damage begins to occur, it can't be repaired. Certain urine tests can help your doctor pick up very early abnormalities. If these are detected, your physician can recommend a course of treatment which may slow or even prevent the development of end-stage renal (kidney) disease requiring a kidney transplant or dialysis.

If your kidneys lose their ability to function, you may experience the following symptoms, which are found in end-stage renal disease:

- Swelling of the ankles, hands, face, or other parts of your body.
- Loss of appetite, accompanied by a metallic taste in your mouth.
- Skin irritations, caused by the buildup of waste products.
- Difficulty thinking clearly.
- Difficulty managing your blood glucose.
- Fatigue, caused by your body's inability to cope with the buildup of fluid and waste materials.

You may not notice all of the above-mentioned symptoms. And they usually don't occur suddenly. In fact, the onset of symptoms generally is gradual. Nonetheless, they do signal loss of kidney function. People in the early stages of kidney damage may experience no symptoms. So to detect kidney problems at an early stage, your doctor will test your urine and blood for the presence of minute amounts of protein and other substances, which are the earliest signs of decreasing kidney function. By identifying and treating the problem early on, the process may be slowed or even stopped, so be sure to ask your doctor if he is performing these tests, and what the results show.

Once damaged, the kidneys usually continue to deteriorate as years go by. Eventually, they could fail completely. When the kidneys are operating at 10 percent capacity or less, you must find other ways to carry out their tasks. This may involve a blood-cleansing method called *dialysis*. There are two types of dialysis. With the first type, *hemodialysis*, the blood is cleansed by a machine at a hospital or clinic or sometimes at home. The blood is circulated through the machine, which removes all impurities and returns it to the patient. The procedure needs to be performed three or four times a week, with each procedure lasting 3 to 5 hours. With the second type, *peritoneal dial-*

ysis, a fluid flows into the body through a tube that has been permanently inserted in the abdomen. This fluid absorbs the wastes and is then drained and replaced by new fluid. This method, which can be done at home, takes about 40 minutes each time and must be repeated three or four times a day.

An alternative to dialysis is *kidney transplantation*. It is a surgical procedure in which the person receives a healthy kidney from a donor (see Figure 17-4). People can live with just one kidney, so this causes little threat to the donor, who is often a close relative of the patient.

Figure 17-4

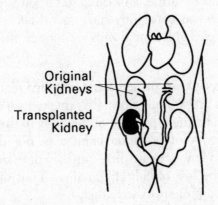

Original Kidneys

Transplanted Kidney

Preventing Kidney Damage

Dealing with kidney damage can take a great deal of energy and effort, and it's in your best interest to do everything to keep your kidneys as healthy as possible. If kidney damage does occur, it cannot be repaired. But there are steps you can take to slow down the progression of the damage.

KEEP YOUR BLOOD SUGAR IN CONTROL. Certain types of kidney damage are linked to poor diabetes control. Therefore, one of the best ways to take care of your kidneys is to keep your blood sugar in the normal range. Monitor your blood sugar regularly. Stick to the meal plans and exercise programs devised by your health-care team.

REDUCE HIGH BLOOD PRESSURE. Keeping your blood pressure at proper levels is also very important. High blood pressure puts further strain on the kidneys and it should be treated promptly with appropriate medication and changes in your diet. Normal blood pressure should have a top number (systolic) no greater than 140, and a bottom number (diastolic) no greater than 90. Learn to check your own blood pressure, record the results, and report any changes to your health-care team. A diet low in sodium may help lower your blood pressure, so ask your dietitian to help you develop a low-sodium meal plan (see guidelines on pages 60–61). Regular exercise and losing excess weight can also reduce blood pressure.

TREAT URINARY TRACT INFECTIONS. Urinary tract infections can damage your kidneys and they should be treated immediately by your physician. Get regular checkups and know the signs of such an infection—cloudy or bloody urine, a burning sensation, frequent urination, or the feeling that you constantly have to urinate. The earlier these infections are detected and treated with antibiotics, the better for the life of your kidneys.

TEST FOR PROTEIN. Your urine should be tested regularly for protein. When the kidneys are working normally, they return the protein to the blood, rather than letting it pass out of the body in the urine. If protein is present in your urine, it means the kidneys are not filtering substances properly. Eating a low-protein diet can ease the kidneys' workload, possibly slowing the loss of kidney function. Your dietitian can show you ways to reduce protein in your diet.

TEST FOR MICROALBUMINURIA. Your doctor should also test your urine periodically for *microalbuminuria*. This test, usually done on the urine sample you leave during a routine medical exam, measures very small amounts of protein in the urine. While the presence of microalbuminuria does not signal the level of problems indicated by the presence of larger amounts of protein (see above), it does suggest that some early kidney damage is occurring. When microalbuminuria is present, your physician may want to start treating you with medication that might help protect your kidneys from further damage. This medication may also be used in people who have high blood pressure. Your physician may prescribe this medication even if you don't have high blood pressure because research shows it may slow kidney damage.

TEST FOR CREATININE. Be sure your doctor tests your blood for *creatinine*, a waste product derived from the activity of your muscles. Normally, your kidneys can remove this substance from your blood. A buildup of creatinine in your blood signals that your kidneys are losing their ability to function normally.

Will these preventive measures really help? Yes! According to recent research studies, whatever you do today to keep your kidneys' functions as "normal" as possible will increase your chances of healthier kidneys in the long run. Good control of diabetes is the key to preventing kidney damage.

THE NERVES

Your nerves also can be damaged by chronic high blood sugar. Called *neuropathy*, it is a condition that can be very debilitating and painful. Neuropathy strikes in many forms. Some people say it feels like walking on pins and needles or walking on steel wool. If your hands are affected, neuropathy may feel like constantly wearing a pair of gloves.

Why does diabetes affect the nerves? Nerves are like electric wires. They are surrounded by a sheath of cells, called Schwann cells, that are like the insulation that covers electric wires. Sugar from the blood can get into the Schwann cells, causing them to swell and squeeze the nerves. The nerves become irritated, often resulting in severe pain.

There are two main types of neuropathy, depending on which nerve cells are damaged. One type is called *sensory neuropathy*, which affects nerves that control sensation in the body. The most common form of sensory neuropathy affects feeling in your legs or hands and is referred to as peripheral neuropathy. The other main type is *autonomic neuropathy*, which affects nerves that control various organs, such as your stomach or urinary tract.

Sensory Neuropathy

If you have diabetes, you may be painfully familiar with sensory nerve damage. It usually affects the extremities—legs, arms, or hands. It also can affect nerves that send signals to your body's skeletal muscles. Symptoms may include numbness, coldness, tingling, or the feeling that you are walking on steel wool. Occasionally, there is pain that feels like tightening bands across the chest or abdomen. Sometimes cold or wet weather makes the condition worse. The pain is often worse at night, making the weight of bedclothes unbearable.

Sensory neuropathy can occur in nearly any nerve. The feeling ranges from minor discomfort to severe pain. Eventually, the pain may disappear—not necessarily because the condition is better, but because the nerves have died! Once dead, the nerves can never grow back and you have lost all sensation at that site. That loss of feeling results in numbness. By maintaining better control of your blood sugar, you can help prevent extensive nerve damage.

If you lose sensation in a certain part of your body, you may face another problem. You may have trouble recognizing minor injuries. For example, you may not feel the development of a blister on your foot, which may then become infected. Or you may unknowingly place your feet in scalding water. The foot bones, too, may suffer because of the lack of feeling. The final result may be the loss of a limb.

Sensory neuropathy may also affect muscles triggered by sensory nerves. Throughout the body, constant tiny electrical impulses travel from your nerves to your muscles. This process normally helps preserve muscle tone. When neuropathy destroys the nerve cells, they cannot stimulate the nearby muscle, resulting in muscle wasting (*amyotrophy*). If this occurs in your thighs, you may experience a painful condition that causes the thigh muscles to decrease in bulk and strength. You may have difficulty rising from a chair or climbing stairs. Your doctor can try to treat this condition with pain relievers and nerve-quieting medications. You also may be advised to increase your physical activity to help restore muscle strength. Recovery usually is slow, so don't expect overnight changes.

If the muscles responsible for raising the foot are weakened, your foot slaps with each step (*foot-drop*). You may be advised to wear a brace, and recovery usually takes place in time. *Charcot foot* is also a problem that can evolve as a result of nerve damage. In this rare condition, the small bones of the foot become misaligned and the foot becomes deformed. If you develop this problem, you may require bed rest or other treatment to keep weight off the affected foot. Patients are often advised to exercise the large muscles of their legs to prevent further muscle wasting. See Chapter 18 for more information on this condition.

Occasionally neuropathy affects a single nerve that operates a muscle or group of muscles. If the muscles of the eye are involved, you might experience double vision. The condition may continue for three to six weeks or more. But in time, most people completely recover. A less common type of sensory neuropathy involves the muscles in the chest or abdomen. The person feels sharp, burning pain that seems to encircle the body. People often mistake this for heart pain. This condition, called *truncal neuropathy*, usually disappears gradually. Of course, any type of chest pain should be evaluated by a doctor. Something else could be wrong.

Autonomic Neuropathy

Autonomic neuropathy affects "involuntary" nerves in the body. These include the nerves that control the actions of the stomach, intestine, esophagus, bladder, penis, and even the circulatory system.

If neuropathy strikes the nerves controlling your digestive tract, you may have trouble processing and disposing of food, a condition called *gastroparesis*. Symptoms include bouts of nausea, vomiting, diarrhea, or constipation. Your doctor can prescribe medications to help with these problems. For nausea and vomiting due to neuropathy, you may be given drugs to increase the motility of your digestive tract and help food move along. Eating smaller, more frequent meals may help lessen the symptoms. You may also be told to decrease the amount of fiber in your diet. For diarrhea, your doctor may prescribe diphenoxylate and atropine (often sold under the brand name Lomotil) or loperamide (Imodium).

Sometimes diabetes damages the nerves that control the contraction of blood vessels. If you have this condition, your blood pressure may fall when you stand or when you sit up from a lying position. When you have been lying down and get up quickly, you may feel weak and dizzy. If severe, this condition, called *orthostatic hypotension*, can be helped by a certain medication that will raise your blood pressure. Of course, this poses a problem if you already have high blood pressure. Your physician will have to carefully balance your prescriptions of pressure-raising and pressure-lowering drugs.

Autonomic neuropathy may also affect your bladder, making it difficult to tell when it is full. To handle this problem, you may find it helpful to get into a regularly scheduled routine of going to the bathroom, perhaps every 2 hours.

Diabetes may affect your sexual function, a complication particularly common to men. Nearly one half of all men with diabetes develop *impotence*, the inability to have or maintain an erection. It is thought that impotence that is caused by diabetes results, in some cases, from damage to the nerves that control the small valves located in the blood vessels leading to and from the penis. These valves regulate the flow of blood into the penis to make it rigid. When nerves are damaged, the man has trouble having or maintaining an erection. For information on ways to treat this problem, see Chapter 16.

For women with diabetes, much less is known about how diabetes may cause specific nerve problems that affect sexual function, although it has been suggested that *vaginal dryness* may occur. Also, high levels of blood sugar may make women more susceptible to *vaginal yeast infections*, which in turn can make intercourse more painful. These topics are also discussed in Chapter 16.

Treating and Preventing Neuropathy

Maintaining blood sugar within normal or near-normal levels is important in treating and preventing neuropathy. In addition, be sure to inform your physician about any tingling or pain as well as numbness or loss of feeling, especially in the body extremities. If you have a loss of sensation in any part of your body, be careful to avoid injuries to that area and check it daily for signs of injury or infection.

To treat sensory neuropathy, your doctor may recommend pain relievers such as aspirin or acetaminophen (Tylenol). To help reduce nerve inflammation, you may be given nonsteroidal antiinflammatory drugs such as naproxen (sold under several brand names, including Naprosyn) or ibuprofen (found in Motrin, Advil, or Nuprin). Nerve irritation may be relieved by drugs such as promazine (Sparine) or amitriptyline (Elavil). These drugs are often known as antidepressants or mood elevators. If these medications are recommended to you, your doctor is not suggesting the problem is in your head. It's just that these drugs in modest doses seem to help people with neuropathy.

Some people find relief by wearing a body stocking or pantyhose to minimize the rubbing effect of clothes. Others are helped by analgesic ointments such as Ben Gay. Relaxation techniques—biofeedback, self-distraction, imagery, and meditation—also benefit some people. If you are suffering from neuropathy, talk to your health-care team about possible treatment options. And remember, most important is to do whatever you can to gain good control of your blood sugar.

BLOOD VESSELS

Complications from diabetes can occur in the blood-vessel system. Also called the cardiovascular system, it is the means by which blood is pumped from your heart and circulated throughout your body. As it circulates, the blood carries nourishment and oxygen to all of your body's tissues. It also removes waste products. In general, problems occur when there is a gradual thickening of the walls of the blood vessels, resulting in poor circulation and other ailments. The common thread in all heart and blood-vessel diseases is blockage of the arteries—either partial or total. The leading cause is *atherosclerosis*, the buildup of plaque deposits in the blood vessels. The disease is common in older people as a result of aging, but it intensifies in people with diabetes.

What does all this mean to a person with diabetes? Research shows that people with diabetes are more likely to develop cardiovascular disease than people who do not have the disease. To date, it is not clearly understood exactly why this happens, but studies suggest that high levels of sugar in the blood can damage the blood vessels. Also, people with diabetes tend to have higher amounts of fats in their blood. This contributes to plaque buildup in the blood vessels, which narrows them and sets the stage for clot formation.

The link between heart disease and diabetes is convincing. Studies show that among people who have had a recent heart attack, one third to one half have had abnormal blood sugar levels, at least temporarily. Researchers have also learned that heart attack is a chief cause of death in people whose diabetes developed after age 30.

Atherosclerosis can progress from a thickening of the blood vessels to a partial or complete blockage, which brings on a number of very serious consequences. Partial blockage of the large coronary arteries that supply blood to the heart may cause chest pains (*angina*) as sections of the heart become damaged from lack of nutrients. If the blood supply is blocked altogether, a heart attack (*myocardial infarction*) may occur. A blockage in the circulation of blood to the brain may cause a stroke. Blockages in the blood vessels that supply blood to the legs and feet can cause pain in the thigh or calf muscles when standing, walking, or exercising. This condition is called *peripheral vascular disease*.

In addition to high blood sugar, other factors increase your risk of developing blood-vessel disease. Being overweight is one risk factor. If you need to lose weight, read Chapter 6. And talk to your health-care team about adjusting your calorie intake and getting more exercise.

Eating foods containing large amounts of saturated fat and cholesterol increases the level of cholesterol in the blood, particularly "bad" cholesterol (see discussion on pages 51–52). This can lead to clogging of the blood vessels, reduced circulation, and an increased risk of cardiovascular disease. A meal plan low in saturated fat and cholesterol is essential, so be sure to consult with your dietitian about these matters.

High blood pressure (*hypertension*) also speeds up the process of atherosclerosis. If you develop high blood pressure, your physician may want you to lose weight and reduce the amount of salt in your diet. If your blood pressure remains high, your physician may treat it aggressively with medications.

Smoking is another factor that increases the risk of blood vessel disease. That's because *nicotine*, the major chemical absorbed by the body from cigarette smoking, narrows or constricts the blood vessels. This is bad news for people with diabetes, who are already at risk for blood-vessel disease. Smoking adds additional risk and is particularly hazardous.

THE SKIN

The skin is the body's largest organ. It serves as your "protective armor," the first line of defense against invading organisms. People with diabetes have the same skin problems as other people, but they also have problems specific to poorly controlled diabetes. One is excessively dry skin, caused by dehydration. This essentially means you do not have enough fluids in your body's tissues, which is often the outcome of poorly controlled diabetes. Dry skin can be treated with a skin lotion containing lanolin and, of course, by getting better control of high blood sugar.

Sometimes "shin spots" appear on the front of the legs. These are quite harmless and nothing to worry about. However, you also have the possibility of getting fungal infections, which are discussed in Chapter 18.

Fatty plaques (*xanthomas*), which are orange-yellow in color, may appear around the eyes or on the shins or elbows. They sometimes are related to high blood levels of cholesterol or triglycerides. You can help this condition disappear with proper diabetes control and by reducing dietary saturated fats and cholesterol (see Chapter 4). Your doctor may also prescribe medications that can lower fat.

The most specific skin problem in people with diabetes is something with a jaw-breaking name—*necrobiosis lipoidica diabeticorum*, usually just called NLD. A relatively harmless condition, it can nevertheless be quite disfiguring. Doctors believe NLD results from an inflammation of the skin in which the skin thins out, becoming discolored and dimpled. What actually is happening is the destruction of the layer of fat in the skin.

For unknown reasons, NLD occurs more in women than in men, generally in the teen years. It is most often found on the front of the legs between the knees and ankles, and first appears as a pink or red discoloration, which later becomes shiny and tight, much like the skin of an apple. Although generally harmless, this condition can be alarming. You can be assured that the discolored areas often improve, although it may take years. The main danger of this condition is that the area may break open, form a sore, and become infected. To hide the blemishes, you can use cosmetics or wear slacks.

There is no satisfactory treatment for NLD. Ointments are generally ineffective, although some cases have improved with cortisone treatment. Skin grafts are sometimes necessary for severe cases, which fortunately are rare. Researchers are experimenting with new treatments. For example, some scientists propose that NLD may be caused by the clumping of platelets, tiny cells that are part of the blood-clotting mechanism, which leads to blockage and inflammation of blood vessels and the beginning of NLD. Some physicians suggest using "anticlumping" medications to slow the progression of the condition. To date, this treatment is still experimental, but there may be hope for the future.

Another condition that is associated with insulin resistance in diabetes is a thickening and darkening of the skin in patchy areas called *acanthosis nigricans*. This is usually a cosmetic problem, but in someone who does not yet have diabetes it may be a clue that you will develop it in the future.

SORTING IT OUT

You should be aware of the wide range of long-term complications that can arise from your diabetes. But don't make the mistake of thinking *all* your medical problems are related to your diabetes. You may be ignoring a completely different problem that needs prompt attention. How can you sort it out? Perhaps you can't—and it's best left to the judgment of your physician. Many people see one doctor for their primary care and a diabetes specialist for their diabetes. This is strongly recommended by organizations like Joslin and the American Diabetes Association. As a general rule, if you are unsure about a particular problem or wondering if it's related to your diabetes, ask a member of your diabetes health-care team.

If you have a new health problem, bring it up when you see your primary-care physician. Don't wait until you see your diabetes specialist. And be sure to see your diabetes specialist *at least* every 6 months, and an ophthalmologist *at least* once a year to check your eyes. Also, plan to work with other members of your health-care team—the nurse educator, dietitian, and others—to solve any specific problems you may have.

The emotional strain of dealing with diabetes and the threat of long-term complications can take a toll. The members of your health-care team can help you personally sort out your feelings. They can also direct you to a specialist who is trained to help you cope emotionally with a lifelong disease. This topic is covered more fully in Chapter 19. Most diabetes centers have support groups in which people share their problems and help each other find solutions. You can also check with the American Diabetes Association, the Juvenile Diabetes Foundation, or local diabetes societies for listings of any groups in your area.

During the past decades, major advances have been made in diagnosing, treating, and preventing the long-term complications of diabetes. Researchers have produced remarkable treatments for eyes, kidneys, nerves, blood-vessel disease, and other problems associated with diabetes. As research continues, you can expect even more improvements in treatments for these problems. But success in the immediate future rests with you and your health-care team. By learning about long-term complications and watching for their signs, you are pivotal in arresting their progress. And by learning how to prevent them—particularly with good diabetes management—you have the promise of a healthier you!

CHAPTER 18

Foot Care and Diabetes

PEOPLE WITH DIABETES have a greater chance of developing foot problems. In fact, they spend more days in the hospital with foot complications than with any other problem. However, many of these complications are preventable. For that reason, your health-care team will ask you to pay special attention to your feet.

Why are you at a higher risk? A combination of the following factors sets the stage for foot trouble:

- People with diabetes often have less sensation in their feet due to nerve damage (*neuropathy*), as discussed in Chapter 17.
- People with diabetes tend to have more narrowing or blockage in their blood vessels, also discussed in Chapter 17.
- Many people with Type II diabetes (non-insulin-dependent) are older or are overweight and can't reach down to properly inspect or care for their feet.
- People who have had diabetes for a long time frequently have eye complications that affect their ability to see where they are setting their feet and to examine their feet adequately.
- People with poorly controlled diabetes have a higher risk for infection because their ability to fight infections is reduced.

SYMPTOMS OF FOOT PROBLEMS

One of the most common problems for people with diabetes is nerve damage that results in a loss of feeling in the feet. For example, you may step on a tack without noticing any pain. Or you may be totally unaware of a severe burn on your feet from walking barefoot on hot pavement. The loss of feeling also makes you unaware of a sore or injury, which can then more easily become infected because you don't take care of the injury.

Another common condition in diabetes is poor circulation. Circulation in the blood vessels deteriorates with age, but the problem is accelerated in people with diabetes. The legs and feet are among the first to be affected, because they are farthest from the heart. Signs of poor circulation include

- Cramps that occur in the legs while walking but go away after resting.
- Slow healing cuts and scratches.
- Redness of your feet when you are sitting, or whiteness when they are propped up on a stool or chair.
- Lack of normal hair growth on the legs and feet.
- Pain in your feet and legs, especially at night, which can be relieved by hanging them over the side of the bed; this is a sign of more advanced disease.

The feet are very vulnerable to infection, due to the nerve and circulation diseases that frequently complicate diabetes, particularly if it is poorly controlled. Infections begin with damage to the skin, which serves as a protective barrier. Once damaged, the barrier is no longer intact and provides an entryway for invading organisms, leading to infection. Damage to your skin can result from an injury, irritation, or foot deformities. Common foot problems include corns and calluses, ingrown toenails, fungal infections (athlete's foot), and sores caused by pressure to the foot, perhaps from poorly fitting shoes.

Unless treated promptly, a foot infection can lead to a chain of events that worsen it with time. In the presence of infection, the body responds with inflammation and swelling, which diminishes the blood flow. Poor circulation decreases the body's ability to get disease-fighting cells to the infection site. Moreover, poor blood sugar control makes these cells less effective in battling the infection. And with neuropathy, you cannot feel the pain of infection. In fact, your nerves may be so dull that you continue to walk on the injured part. The situation is particularly dangerous when there is pus or drainage from a sore and the foot is red hot and swollen. If you ever have this problem, *go to the emergency room at once.* You need the immediate care of a medical doctor to stop the infection—before the tissue dies. Treatment is crucial if you are to save your foot or toe.

Another problem that may develop is *Charcot foot.* This is a condition that affects approximately 1 of every 700 people who have diabetes, and it is usually limited to those who have moderate to severe loss of feeling in their feet. Charcot foot is more common among people who are overweight, but it can also occur in thin people. No one is quite sure how Charcot foot begins. However, it is thought to be caused by either an incidental trauma or a twist of the foot which injures some of the ligaments that support the arch of the foot. Once the ligaments have been damaged, the bones begin grinding against one another and the arch may collapse. The damage often goes unnoticed because the person has already lost feeling in his foot. With the collapse of the bones in the arch, the weight is distributed differently along the sole of the foot, causing increased pressure points and irritation, which may lead to sores and infection.

If your foot swells without explanation and is warm to the touch with no apparent break in the skin, you may have Charcot foot. When these symptoms occur, be sure your physician or foot doctor (podiatrist) examines your foot. Charcot foot must be differentiated from the red-hot swollen foot caused by infection. With infection, you should go to the emergency room immediately.

Rest is the primary treatment for Charcot foot. Depending on the severity of the damage, no weight should be placed on your foot for 8–16 weeks. Permanent foot deformities can be avoided if the condition is diagnosed and treated early.

GUIDELINES FOR DAILY FOOT CARE

To minimize the risk of foot problems from diabetes, it's important to follow a daily routine of foot care and inspection.

Wash Your Feet

Wash, but do not soak, your feet in warm, soapy water each day. Soaking softens the skin and makes it more susceptible to infection. *Never* use hot water. Always test the temperature of the water with your elbow. This will prevent burning your feet if you have nerve damage and cannot feel the water temperature. Use a mild hand soap to wash your feet. Rinse your feet well after washing, and dry them carefully, especially between the toes.

Examine Your Feet

Each day, look at your feet in good light. Be sure you examine the bottom of your feet. If you cannot bend over to see the bottom, place a hand mirror on the floor and hold each foot over it. If your eyesight is poor, have someone examine your feet for you. Look for areas of dryness or breaks in the skin, especially around the toenails and between the toes. Notify your doctor immediately about sores or infections that do not seem to be healing properly. Redness, swelling, and increased warmth are signs of infection.

Care for Your Skin

After washing and examining your feet, lubricate your feet to prevent dryness. Use a moisture-restoring cream such as Nivea, Eucerin, or Alpha-Keri. Creams are better than lotions because they hold moisture in the skin for a longer time. Begin applying the cream at your heels and work toward your toes. Avoid getting cream between the toes; the skin could wear away, leading to infection. Do not use perfumed lotions because they contain alcohol, which dries rather than lubricates. Do not put any lotions or creams between your toes. If your feet perspire, use talcum, baby powder, or a mild foot powder to absorb the moisture. Do not allow the powder to cake between the toes.

File Your Toenails

File your nails with a diamond-type (emery) board. Never use scissors or clippers because you might cut yourself, leading to infection. Don't file your nails shorter than the ends of your toes. Shape them according to the contours of your toes and the toes next to them. If you have poor vision, have a friend or podiatrist trim your nails when needed. Consult a foot doctor for ingrown toenails or fungal nail infections that lead to discoloration and thickening. These conditions need expert care.

Care for Corns, Calluses, Blisters, and Warts

Corns and calluses can increase pressures on the feet and are signs of potential ulcers. If neglected, they can lead to irritation and possible infection. Properly fitting shoes can relieve and prevent these thickened areas of skin. After washing your feet, rub any corns or calluses hard with a towel. Use a moisture-restoring cream to soften them. Do not tear off loose skin, and never use corn- or callus-removal products. Don't cut corns or calluses—do not perform bathroom surgery! Watch for discoloration on or around corns and calluses, which could indicate a more serious problem such as an ulcer beneath the skin. Because of the potential for foot ulcers, corns and calluses should be examined regularly by a foot doctor, who may decide to thin or remove them.

Blisters should be treated with antiseptic. Warts are difficult to treat and may disappear if left alone. Like calluses, plantar warts (on the soles) lead to point pressure and may ulcerate. If a wart begins to spread or causes you pain when walking, consult your physician or podiatrist.

Wear Good Footwear

In addition to daily foot care, you should be concerned about your footwear. Buy shoes that protect and cover your feet and have been properly fitted. Don't go barefoot (especially on the beach) or wear sandals, clogs, or "flip-flops"—your feet need more protection. Make sure your shoes allow room for your toes to rest in their natural positions; avoid pointed shoes that squeeze your toes together. When you wear slippers around your house, be sure they are sturdy enough to prevent stubbing your toes. Always check inside your shoes for foreign objects before putting them on. Break new shoes in gradually to prevent blisters from forming. If you have nerve damage, change your shoes and socks every three or four hours.

Wear Proper Socks and Stockings

Cotton and wool socks and stockings are best, but any machine-washable hosiery is okay. Wear a clean pair each day. If your feet sweat, change your socks several times a day. Make sure they are the correct size and free of seams and darns. Never wear socks or stockings with constricting tops; these can decrease the circulation in your legs. Constricting garters and girdles also should be avoided. Check your socks for drainage, which may be your first sign of a new ulcer or blister.

Exercise Your Feet

Walking is the best exercise for your feet, providing your shoes fit properly. Walking helps the circulation in the feet. After exercising, be sure to check your feet for signs of irritation or blister formation.

Avoid Injury from Heat and Cold

Don't let your feet get too hot. Avoid sunburn, walking barefoot on hot pavement, electric heating pads, hot-water bottles, and bath water that is too hot (test it first with a bath thermometer). Cold and frostbite also can harm foot tissue, so be sure to be extra protective of your feet in cold weather. Beware of exposed radiators and steam rooms or saunas as sources of potential burns.

FIRST-AID TREATMENT

Once in a while, something will happen to your feet, so it's important to know the basic guidelines for first-aid care.

Cuts and Scratches

Treat cuts and scratches promptly. Wash the affected area with warm water and soap. *Do not soak.* You may apply a mild antiseptic such as ST/37 or Bactine. Never use strong antiseptics such as iodine, Betadine, mercurochrome, boric acid, Epsom salts, creosol, or carbolic acid. Cover the affected area with a dry sterile dressing and paper tape or a Telfa bandage. Do not use adhesive tape or Band-Aids, as they may cause allergic reactions or irritations. Do not apply heat treatments such as a hot-water bottle or heating pad to the cut or scratch. Stay off your feet as much as possible and call your physician if the affected areas do not improve within 24 to 30 hours. If red, swollen areas develop or a yellowish drainage occurs, contact your physician immediately. Do not assume the condition has improved just because there is no pain.

Athlete's Foot

Athlete's foot is caused by a fungus that grows in a warm, moist setting. Symptoms are itching, tiny blisters, and the scaling of skin between the toes or on the soles of the feet. If these symptoms appear, consult your physician to make sure it is athlete's foot, rather than some other skin problem. Since the fungus of athlete's foot grows in a warm, moist setting, you should wash and carefully dry your feet and change your socks or stockings more than once a day. Feet that perspire heavily are more likely to get athlete's foot, so keep your feet as dry as possible. If your skin is too moist, apply talcum, baby powder, or a mild foot powder to absorb the moisture. Changing socks will also "wick" moisture away from the skin. Treat athlete's foot with an over-the-counter antifungal product such as Lotrimin, Tinactin, or Desinex. Avoid sneakers or boots. Do not use any other remedies without the consent of your physician or podiatrist. If these measures don't work within 7 to 10 days, stronger prescription drugs may be needed, so consult your doctor.

Ten Rules for Foot Care

1. Never soak your feet!
2. Never apply heat of any kind to your feet.
3. Never cut your toenails—file them.
4. Never wear shoes that do not fit.
5. Never go barefoot.
6. Never use strong medicines on your feet.
7. Never allow corns or calluses to go untreated.
8. Never perform bathroom surgery on your feet.
9. Never keep your feet too moist or too dry.
10. Never assume that the sensation and circulation in your feet are normal. Instead, treat your feet as though they are ripe for trouble—which they are!

Today, you have every reason to be hopeful about preventing and treating foot problems. Again, good management of your blood sugar is essential to the health of your circulatory and nervous systems. The longer these symptoms stay healthy, the less chance you have of developing serious foot infections.

It's also comforting to know that damaged feet that once would have been lost are now being saved. This success is due to a number of factors—better care of diabetes, the use of antibiotics, and improved surgical techniques. For example, clogged blood vessels that cannot transport blood drawn to the legs and feet can often be replaced by grafting blood vessels from other parts of the body or using synthetic vessels. There are also drugs which increase the flexibility of the membranes of red blood cells, allowing them to pass through partially clogged arteries. Of course, the best strategy is prevention. Exercise can improve circulation; with daily inspection and care of your feet—and by keeping your diabetes in control—you can help prevent many foot problems, and keep those that develop from becoming limb-threatening.

Part Six

LIVING WITH DIABETES

CHAPTER 19

Coping with Diabetes

IF YOU HAVE DIABETES, you face a wide range of special challenges. The first of these challenges is physical. You have to learn how your body works—how it uses the food you eat for energy—and how diabetes affects these bodily functions. You need to conscientiously practice a variety of treatment and monitoring procedures to help you avoid high and low blood sugar and the threats they pose to your health.

Other challenges you face are emotional. You need to cope with how diabetes makes you feel—and how you feel about having diabetes. You and your family will inevitably have concerns, anxieties, and fears as you live with this condition over the weeks, months, and years. But most people find that over time, they are remarkably resilient and able to deal effectively with their diabetes. But it's always important to remember that there are a number of ways diabetes can affect your emotions—and a number of ways that your emotions can affect your diabetes.

COMMON CHALLENGES

When you have diabetes, it's easy to believe you are the only person who feels a certain way. It's easy to become reluctant about sharing your feelings with others. However, it's important to realize you are not alone. Many other people are struggling with the same feelings and emotions you are.

Blood Sugar and Emotions

Both high and low blood sugar can cause obvious changes in your mood. For example, low blood sugar can make you nervous or irritable. By contrast, high blood sugar can make you feel very tired, which can cause you to feel listless or depressed. The effects of high and low blood sugar on the emotions vary from person to person. The effect on your emotions of the varying sugar levels is more likely to be the result of feeling poorly because of the high and low sugar values than any direct effect that the sugar has on the mood control center of the brain itself. Don't fall into the trap of attributing all of your feelings—particularly negative ones—to your blood sugar levels. Remember, you actually may be responding to other circumstances in your personal life.

Try to distinguish between feelings related to blood sugar levels and those caused by other factors. Blaming all your feelings on your diabetes may prevent you from uncovering the true source of your distress, and that can keep you from solving a problem and feeling happier. It can also be frustrating to family members and friends, because it prevents them from interacting and sharing honest feelings with you. If you are upset or depressed about something, try to identify the source of the problem. This strategy can help you find the right road to a solution.

Stress and Diabetes Control

People with diabetes often feel that the stresses of everyday life can affect their blood sugar. There is, in fact, scientific evidence that stress may cause blood sugar to either rise or fall. Research also shows that some people with diabetes may be more sensitive than others to the way stress affects blood sugar.

You may find that emotional stress from tense circumstances at home or work can raise or lower your blood sugar. There are two basic ways this can happen. On one hand, stress hormones can be released in your body, causing blood sugar levels to fluctuate. On the other hand, stressful situations can also cause you to change key behaviors that upset your daily routine, making it harder to care for your diabetes. To offset the effects of stress, you may wish to try counseling. Many diabetes centers have professional counselors who are trained to help people with diabetes deal with stresses that can impinge on good diabetes management. It is valuable for any counselor you see to have some background in diabetes. It will also be helpful for your counselor to speak with the members of your treatment team. Exercise and relaxation techniques can also help some people handle stress more effectively.

As you deal with the care of both your body and emotions, it's important to avoid isolating yourself from other people. At times, you may be tempted to withdraw because you feel that people unfamiliar with diabetes cannot possibly understand your experience. While it may be true that some people will not understand, many others will. Seeking the support of your family and friends and making connections with other people who have diabetes can be helpful. In particular, it's important to share your concerns with your doctor and other professionals on your health-care team. Be sure to include members of your family in visits with your health-care team to increase communication between you and your family and your health-care providers.

You may also find it helpful to participate in a diabetes support group in which people share how they have addressed the unique challenges of their diabetes. Your health-care team and local chapter of the American Diabetes Association can tell you where these groups meet in your area.

UNIQUE STRESSES OF DIABETES

People with diabetes have unique day-to-day stresses. Below are a few of the more common difficulties people with diabetes have told clinicians at Joslin they face. You may find that you can identify with many or all of them, which is only normal, because diabetes affects people's bodies and feelings in very similar ways. What will be different is how people cope with these issues. Diabetes is a full-time job that requires persistent effort and commitment. That's why we recommend that you don't "fly solo." Ask for the support and help of family members and friends as well as your physician and other health-care professionals.

Chronic Condition

Diabetes is a *chronic* disorder, something that never goes away. It requires daily care and attention, and for many people, that can be emotionally draining, particularly if there are other stresses in their lives. One person describes it this way: "It's not so much the rolling of a boulder up a hill, it's the stone in the shoe."

Diabetes is all about learning what to do, then doing it day after day despite changing circumstances. How do you deal with this "irksome stone"? First of all, there's nothing wrong with admitting that you hate diabetes. That's right, *hate* it. No one could expect you to do otherwise. At the same time, you must *tolerate* it enough to convert your emotional energy into taking good care of yourself. Such honesty about your feelings will help you strike a healthy emotional balance. You will be able to deal much better with your everyday care.

Practically everyone who is diagnosed with diabetes goes through various emotional stages. For the first few days, you were probably *shocked* by the news, perhaps overwhelmed and confused by it all. You then may have gone through a stage of *denial*, thinking that you didn't really have diabetes, or if you did, it wasn't really a big deal. In fact, some people continue to deny the seriousness of having diabetes for a long time, facing the reality of the situation only when complications set in after many years of poorly controlling their blood sugar.

Another common reaction is *fear* or *anxiety* over the possibility that diabetes will lead to long-term problems with your eyes, kidneys, nerves, or other body systems. Because these complications are more likely to occur with poor diabetes control, it's vitally important that you reach the stage of *accepting* your condition as soon as possible. By accepting the realities of diabetes and its proper care, you can begin to gain mastery over this chronic condition. A growing understanding that good blood sugar control can prevent or minimize complications will give you some feeling of control over your own future health. Of course, there will still be days when you feel distressed and overwhelmed by your diabetes, even after you've accepted the realities of having it.

"Invisible" Nature

Diabetes is an invisible condition, a disease that generally remains hidden. If you walk into a room, you can easily spot someone with a runny nose from a cold, but you can't tell who has diabetes. This invisibility factor can bring internal and interpersonal conflict. On one hand, you feel the "same" as other people, with many of the same desires and needs. You may love to eat sweets and thrive on independence. On the other hand, you feel "different." Unlike people who don't have diabetes, you have to watch what you eat and sacrifice some of your independence to take care of your health. Coping with this tension—simultaneously feeling the same and different—can take some work. To put these feelings in perspective, talk them out with your family members and health-care team.

The hidden nature of diabetes makes it "a disease in the absence of illness." In other words, if you are keeping your diabetes somewhat in control, you may not experience any immediate symptoms, even though subtle changes may be occurring throughout your body that can lead to long-term complications. This lack of visible signs can lead to lapses in your treatment program. After all, it's easy to remember to take a decongestant when you have a stuffy nose. It's not so easy to follow a meal plan, exercise regularly, monitor your blood, and take medication when there are no apparent warning signs. You may find it hard to keep your diabetes program on track as a result. Others may find it difficult to remember your need to keep to a schedule or watch what you eat.

Staying with your treatment program requires concentration. You'll often need to think about when you ate or exercised; you'll need to remember to test your blood sugar, and take your diabetes pills or insulin. You will need to develop a routine, something that's easier for some people to do than others. Adapting to a new lifestyle can take discipline and a lot of patience, qualities that do not come easily to many people. Be patient. Set realistic goals that are achievable. Over time, you can improve your care, step by step.

Frustration

Diabetes can cause frustration and anger. At times, you may be upset that you have diabetes in the first place. You may feel overwhelmed as you struggle to learn the basic things you need to know to care for your condition. There may be days that caring for your diabetes seems to get in the way of your job, your personal relationships, and just plain having fun. Feeling angry or frustrated, you may slack off on your eating plan, exercise, medication, or monitoring. In fact, experts have identified more than 250 factors that can interfere with following a treatment program—everything from blaming the weather to accusing other people.

How can you deal with frustration? One way is by realizing that everyone with diabetes has good days and bad days. There will be times when you follow your treatment plan and do *not* see the results you hoped for. There will be times and temptations that make it hard to stick with your treatment plan. At a recent workshop for people with diabetes, the discussion leader asked, "What's the biggest thing that gets in the way of sticking to your treatment program?" Without hesitation, everyone in the group shouted, "Food!"

So if you're having trouble with a meal plan, you're certainly not alone. The group also pointed to other major hurdles—dealing with other people's schedules and traveling with diabetes. Sound familiar? You, too, have probably faced these hurdles. To manage your care, you may have to change how you feel about your diabetes and how you can cope when things don't go right. You may get frustrated when you're seemingly doing everything possible to control your blood sugar, but you're not getting good results. That may cause you to ask, "What's the use?" And you may get despondent or angry, taking it out on yourself or other people. You may be tempted to abandon your program.

You need to realize that you will have days of unexplained high or low blood sugar. Also, that it's hard to stay motivated over a long period of time. Be honest about how you feel about this lifelong commitment. In fact, many of the ways you choose to cope with these feelings will require this type of honesty—a clear assessment of the task before you and how you will face occasional disappointments and failures. At those times, rather than throwing in the towel, try to see your diabetes treatment as a long stretch of highway. Once in a while you may veer off the road onto the gravel shoulder, or run out of gas or get a flat tire. But with the help of your health-care team, family, and other people with diabetes, you can get back on the road.

Unpredictability

Diabetes can be very unpredictable. It varies from person to person. Its impact on your body often changes over time, requiring adjustments as you get older. It can change with physical stresses, such as being sick. There even are moments when a sudden change in your blood sugar will occur for no apparent reason. As one person with diabetes put it, "It's just one crazy thing after another." Such unpredictability can be very unsettling, and people can become so anxious about experiencing something like a low-blood-sugar reaction that they may stay home as much as possible, avoiding restaurants or not traveling as much as they would like. Or they may keep blood sugar levels on the "high side" most of the time to avoid having a low-blood-sugar reaction.

To cope with the unpredictable nature of diabetes, it's important to learn as much as possible about your condition. That way, you'll be prepared for high or low blood sugar (see Chapters 11 and 12), what to do on sick days (Chapter 13), how to eat at restaurants (Chapter 20), and how to travel with diabetes (Chapter 22). By being prepared to deal with a variety of situations, you will feel more at ease. Indeed, you'll discover that much of life can go on as before.

A Paradox

Diabetes is a medical problem that must come first in your life. Yet you don't want it to take over your life, and that can raise a host of questions. Are you well or sick? Master or victim? In control or helpless?

Optimistic or pessimistic? Independent or dependent? The way you respond to these questions will depend, in many ways, on your personal characteristics and how you approach life in general. Coping with the paradox of diabetes—it's No. 1 and it's not No. 1—takes emotional honesty, maturity, and support. But by sorting it out, you will be better able to manage your diabetes. Yes, your treatment program will be of utmost importance. But your diabetes has never been and never will be *you*. You are a person with many qualities—feelings, thoughts, and skills that you can use to find personal fulfillment as well as to make contributions to your family, job, and community. By defining yourself in this positive way, your diabetes care becomes a means to an end. Your care is a way to maintain your health so that you're able to be who you really are!

Hope for the Future

It is only natural that once your diabetes was diagnosed, you became concerned about your future. After all, you probably have heard about the possibility of serious complications developing in people who have had diabetes for many years. You may know someone with eye disease or even blindness due to diabetes. You may have heard about people who have had a foot or leg amputated or whose kidneys failed from the effects of poorly controlled diabetes. Naturally, this can make you concerned and anxious, and cause you to question what the future will be like.

Various complications do occur in some people with long-standing, poorly controlled diabetes. However, it must be emphasized again that there is every reason for hope. Research shows that intensive treatment and monitoring procedures—which help you maintain good control of your blood sugar levels—can help prevent, delay, or reduce the severity of complications.

While there is no guarantee that every person will bypass the complications of diabetes, such problems are much less likely to occur if you maintain good blood sugar control. In the Diabetes Control and Complications Trial, physicians followed the progress of people who used "intensive diabetes therapy." These people used multiple doses of insulin each day and maintained tight control of their diabetes by frequently testing their blood sugar throughout the day and adjusting their insulin doses accordingly. Those who had no eye problems at the beginning of the 10-year study had a 76 percent lower chance of having developed signs of eye disease at the end of the study. Those who followed intensive therapy had a 35 percent reduction in the risk of mild protein leakage into the urine (*microalbuminuria*). In addition, intensive therapy reduced the risk of developing nerve disease (*neuropathy*) by 70 percent. Some people on intensive therapy did experience more episodes of serious low-blood-sugar reactions and weight gain. However, the primary finding of the study was that any improvement in blood sugar control was linked to a clear reduction in risk of complications.

Such success stories abound, and they can help motivate you to stay on track with your program. You may wish to consider ways to improve your diabetes control, such as intensive diabetes therapy. You might also like to meet people who are successfully managing diabetes with intensive therapy. Of course, if you decide to embark on this form of care, you will need the help of specialists skilled in intensive therapy.

BE OPEN ABOUT YOUR DIABETES

Some people try to keep their diabetes a secret. They believe if people find out about their condition, they will be considered "different" and will become the object of some type of special attention. They worry about being denied promotions by employers or becoming distanced from friends and acquaintances. Some of these concerns are legitimate. There are people who do not understand diabetes and need to learn more about it. Furthermore, there are employers who are unfamiliar with diabetes and may refuse to employ or promote a person who has it. Therefore, it is unrealistic to say this is a groundless concern.

On the other hand, not letting others know you have diabetes also has its difficulties. You may feel tense and isolated as you try to care for your diabetes while hiding it from the people around you. Letting others know about your condition can bring about the positive support that is so important in dealing with your diabetes. For safety reasons, someone who works closely with you needs to know how to help you in case your blood sugar drops and you have a low-blood-sugar reaction.

Family members, friends, and fellow employees can offer encouragement as you strive to follow an eating program, exercise regularly, take medications, and monitor your condition. Some people with diabetes ask a friend or family member to learn along with them as they work at mastering the art of managing diabetes. They then have a partner who can share their disappointments and victories—and also help in time of need.

KEYS TO SUCCESS

The following checklist highlights ways that you may find helpful in dealing with your diabetes. Review this list on a regular basis, refocusing your feelings and thoughts as other circumstances in your life change.

- *Develop self-awareness.*
  Identify factors that can personally interfere with managing your diabetes. Are you tempted to eat fatty foods? Is it inconvenient to test your blood sugar at school or work? Do you frequently eat out at restaurants? Does your working style cause you to lose track of time? By concentrating on major stumbling blocks to your diabetes care, you will be better able to find ways around them.

- *Be self-reliant.*
  Don't place a lot of responsibility on other people. You essentially are responsible for your diabetes care and overall health. Learn the importance of meal planning, exercise, medications, and testing your blood sugar.

- *Manage stress.*
  Identify factors in your life that cause tension, wear you down, or make you anxious. Work with your health-care team to reduce these stresses.

- *Be prepared.*
  Unlike people who don't have diabetes, you may have to plan out aspects of your day. Also, you need to be ready to handle occasional high and low blood sugar. Being prepared can help you feel more at ease and in control.

- *Set achievable goals.*
  With the help of your health-care team, set practical goals. Approach your diabetes care in a step-by-step manner. Over the years, you will gradually improve in your understanding and techniques.

- *Be realistic.*
  You're not always going to be in great control of your diabetes. You will have good days and bad days. When you occasionally fail, don't dwell on it. Simply try to pick up and continue on without guilt or blame.

- *Ask for support.*

  Tell your family and friends what their support means to you. Define the boundaries of what is personally helpful (something that is supportive to one person may not be supportive to another). Tell family and friends specific ways they can help you follow your treatment program. Bring family members with you to meet with your health-care team. This can be a very constructive way to include them in your support network.

CHAPTER 20

Eating on Special Occasions

MUCH OF YOUR DIABETES care is centered around your eating plan—the foods you eat, coordinated with your exercise program and medication schedule. When you're at home, school, or work, you can develop a routine to take this all into account. But what about when you eat at a restaurant? Or at someone else's house? With a little extra planning and foresight, you can enjoy meals away from home.

But it should be pointed out that one of the most enjoyable aspects of eating out has absolutely nothing to do with food. It's the pleasure of spending time with people important to you. By focusing on the social element of the dining-out experience, you will develop a healthier mind-set. Part of that mind-set is to adapt to the unexpected—food that isn't prepared right, slow service, or the temptation to eat off-limits foods. If the unexpected happens, your meal will still be enjoyable because you already have decided that the most important part of eating out is to enjoy the company of your friends and family.

Of course, eating good foods should still remain high on your list. Even though you are away from your own kitchen, you can still manage your diet. By adapting the guidelines you've learned for managing your diabetes at home, you can develop a strategy for eating out.

CHOOSING A RESTAURANT

Look Carefully

If possible, choose a restaurant that offers a wide selection of broiled and baked foods, such as fish and poultry. Many restaurants now pinpoint items on their menus that are "heart-healthy," foods that are lower in fat, cholesterol, and sodium. Avoid restaurants that offer only large portions of fatty meats and fried foods. This eating-out strategy will help prevent health problems associated with a high-fat diet and will also help if you are trying to shed excess pounds.

Reach a Compromise

If you are part of the group choosing the restaurant, don't be afraid to speak up. Communicate in a clear and positive way. Perhaps you can reach a compromise by going to a restaurant that offers something for everyone—a T-bone steak for your friend and stir-fry chicken for you.

Scout It Out

Perhaps the choice of restaurant has already been made. If you're unfamiliar with the restaurant, call ahead to determine what it offers. Ask if you can request special preparation of foods. May I have baked fish instead of fried? Can you put the sauces on the side? Will you omit high-sodium seasonings? Restaurants are in business to attract and keep customers, so most will be happy to meet your needs. You may find it helpful to decide what you will order during this scouting call. Then when you go out with your friends, you'll be all set.

Danger Ahead: All-You-Can-Eat!

You may believe an all-you-can-eat smorgasbord is a good option. After all, you will be able to see the food, determine how it is prepared, and serve your own portions. If you have fantastic self-control, this strategy may work. But remember, these places are billed as "all you *can* eat," not "all you *should* eat." Most people at smorgasbords are tempted to pile far too much food on their plates—a particular problem if you are trying to lose weight as part of your diabetes program. The food all looks so good that it's hard to resist.

Salad bars pose a similar temptation. If you stick to fresh vegetables and low-calorie dressings, you'll do fine. You may want to experiment with lemon juice or a flavored vinegar for your dressing. But watch out for the cheese, eggs, potato salad, gelatins, and high-fat salad dressings.

Call Your Host

If you've been invited to eat at someone's home, you may want to call a day or so ahead and ask your host to set aside small portions of food for you—the meat portion without gravy, or the vegetables without butter. It is far less embarrassing for a host to make slight adjustments during food preparation than to find out too late!

TIMING IT RIGHT

Meal timing can be very important to people with diabetes. When you take insulin, it peaks at a certain time in your bloodstream. If your meal is delayed, you run the risk of having a low-blood-sugar reaction because the insulin keeps working, whether you eat or not. Some of the early signs of an insulin reaction are shakiness, increased sweating, and nervousness, all of which certainly would put a damper on the occasion. Here are some ways that will help you stick to your "insulin clock."

Speak Up

The key—whether at home or away—is to time your meals around your insulin program, or time your insulin program around your meals. It may require you to become more assertive, so don't hesitate to speak up when your friends or relatives are discussing a time to eat. They certainly will understand your needs.

Perhaps you've been invited to someone's house for dinner. If your host asks you to suggest a time, pick a time close to your normal meal hour. Remember, good hosts are trying to make their guests as comfortable as possible. You won't always have control over your eating schedule. Maybe it's unclear when the meal will be served—a question that can be easily answered with a brief phone call.

Plan for Delays

Perhaps your host has already set the dinner time, for example, on a wedding invitation. If you discover the meal is scheduled more than 2 hours after your normal eating time, plan to make adjustments. Here are some options:

- *"Flip-flopping."* Switch the times of your snack and the meal. Flip-flopping your snack and meal may interfere slightly with your normal cycle of using insulin, but it's much better than not eating at all. For example, if you have Type I diabetes (insulin-dependent), the snack will provide nutrients that can be used by some of the insulin that begins to peak after your regularly scheduled "premeal" injection. In fact, even if you plan to eat your meal on time, a small snack before dinner will help guard against unexpected delays—your table is not ready, or the service is slow. Just remember to count the snack as part of your total calorie intake. If you have Type II diabetes (non-insulin-dependent) and are trying to lose weight, a small snack will help control your appetite. When dinner finally is served, you'll be less likely to overeat.
- *Adjust Your Medication.* If you know your meal will be delayed a long time, you may consider adjusting your medication. For example, if you normally take a short-acting type of insulin before meals, it will enter the bloodstream about 30 minutes later and will reach its maximum effect 2 to 4 hours later. If you are eating out, you may want to change the time you take your regular (short-acting) insulin to about 30 minutes prior to eating. This, of course, may mean that you will have to bring your insulin and syringe with you to the restaurant. If you use diabetes pills, which increase the body's sensitivity to insulin, you may want to adjust the timing of your medication to the time of the meal. Check with a member of your health-care team before doing so.

Timing Your Exercise

Exercise is important to people with diabetes, because it helps maintain blood sugar within a normal range. Blood sugar levels are usually lowest before a meal. If you exercise before eating, your blood sugar may plunge even lower. So if possible, exercise after eating. In fact, exercise can help you regulate your blood sugar after eating out. If you think you may have eaten too much at a restaurant, take a brisk walk afterward to reduce your blood sugar level. For more information on the timing of exercise, see Chapter 5.

What's Best for You

Perhaps you're more comfortable eating out at the lunch hour, rather than at dinner. After all, you'll probably find smaller portions, which will help prevent overeating, and something else that's always welcome—lower prices!

Maybe you tend to overeat at restaurants, no matter what the time of day. If so, try to limit the frequency of eating out. You know yourself best, so be honest. It may mean fewer times out, but overall, you are practicing healthier eating habits. If your job or schedule requires that you eat out frequently at lunchtime, order a salad with lean meats and low-calorie dressing, or a fresh turkey sandwich with lettuce and tomato.

WISE MENU CHOICES

If you use an exchange meal plan, converting your meal plan into foods offered on the menu means computing "exchanges"—foods that you can use to meet the milk, vegetable, fruit, bread/starch, meat, and fat choices in your meal plan. If you are a seasoned meal planner, this is not difficult. You've been learning how to make these decisions for many years as you planned your meals at home. Following are some tips that will help those using exchange meal plans convert your plan into a healthy restaurant meal. (Many of the suggestions presented here are useful for those using other types of eating plans.) Later in this chapter, you'll find a sample lunch menu that shows you how to size up your choices.

Carry a Pocket-Sized Meal-Plan Card

On pages 275–276 there is a sample of a small meal-plan card that you can copy and carry with you in your wallet or purse. Unless you have memorized your meal plan, fill out this card and take it with you when eating out. In some cases, you may already be familiar with the menus and have figured out your exchanges. Or you may have called ahead and planned your choices. If you're satisfied with that decision, you are ready to order. Just keep the menu closed. You will be less likely to be tempted to order something else.

Use Food-Exchange Lists

To convert the foods on the menu to your meal plan, use a food-exchange list (see Appendix: Food Choice Lists). Perhaps you have a good idea how to categorize a wide variety of foods. If not, carry a list with you, perhaps an abbreviated list of foods that you typically eat at restaurants.

Ask the Waiter

At home, you may stick to rather simple cooking. But when eating out, it's more fun to try "fancy" fare, which often is described in unfamiliar terms. You may have to ask the waiter or chef some specific questions, for example, "What is blackened?" (marinated and blackened on a grill, often found in Cajun cuisine).

Prepare Ahead

Better yet, prepare in advance for your restaurant meal by learning how certain dishes are cooked. Check a cookbook or restaurant guide written for people on special diets, comparing food exchanges listed for specific types of food. You'll discover that all chicken breasts are not created equal. For example, a 4-ounce serving of teriyaki chicken breast (marinated in teriyaki sauce and grilled) is a good low-fat choice, but chicken Kiev (chicken breast stuffed with butter and cheese, breaded, deep fried, and topped with butter sauce) is high in fat and should be avoided.

Choose the Entree

When making menu choices, you may want to begin by picking the entree. This portion of your meal is often the greatest source of calories and fat. Look for good low-fat choices, such as fish and poultry (ask the chef to remove the skin before cooking). Read how the food is prepared. If the menu isn't clear on this point, ask the waiter. Avoid the "hidden" fats that come with foods fried in butter or oils. Also find out how the food is served. A low-fat choice like turkey breast can quickly become "fatty" when a rich sauce or gravy is poured on top. Some sauces may be low-fat but contain sugar, such as a sweet-sour sauce. If sautéed in wine, the meat is usually within low-fat guidelines (see "Thumbs Up" list later in this chapter). Whenever possible, ask that the sauce be served on the side. You can always have a taste, but you don't need your food swimming in it!

Restaurant portions are often large, and entrees are often high in calories from protein. For those reasons, you may not want to eat the entire entree yourself. Perhaps you could share this part of your meal with someone else at your table. Another suggestion is to order individual items from the lists of appetizers, soups, salads, and breads. You may be more familiar with these foods, which can be creatively "packaged" into a good solid meal. A sample meal: shrimp cocktail, chicken vegetable soup, chef salad.

Select Other Courses

Most restaurants tend to offer more calories in a meal than most people need. To stick to your eating plan, you may wish to pass by one course entirely. If your meal includes an appetizer, avoid those that are fried. Also avoid foods prepared with heavy dairy products (for example, a sauce made with sour cream or cheese). Good choices are broth-based soups or a small glass of tomato juice.

For your salad, a tossed green lettuce salad supplies bulk that can help you feel full—a good way to not overeat. But be careful about the added carbohydrates and fats found in many salad dressings. Ask for the dressing on the side and use only a small portion. You could also request low-calorie dressings, lemon wedges, or vinegar.

Most American restaurants offer potato or rice with an entree. Steamed rice is a good low-fat choice. A baked potato is also low-fat, but be sure to ask for your condiments on the side. Avoid the fats found in butter and sour cream. To add zest to your potato without the calories, add seasonings like pepper, chives, or mustard. Be aware the potatoes that are fried, au gratin, and scalloped are all higher in fat.

Push Away the Breads

While waiting for an order, you may have the habit of reaching for the breadsticks or rolls on the table. If you calculated the table breads into your meal plan, there's no problem. If you didn't account for them and you have trouble resisting the added calories, place the breads out of reach or ask the waiter to remove them from the table.

Eyeball the Portions

Whenever you go to a restaurant, particularly for the first time, one of the "great unknowns" is how large the portions will be. You'll do a better job estimating restaurant portions if you first have practiced portion control at home. Use standard measuring cups, spoons, and a small scale to develop your ability to judge the right portion size. Size them up carefully at home. At the restaurant, when your order arrives, eyeball the portion size and mentally compare it with servings at home. If it looks large, leave a few bites on your plate. Better yet, immediately place the unneeded portion on a side plate, perhaps offering "a taste" of your dish to others who considered ordering it themselves. And don't forget the system restaurants have long used to help you with portion control—the doggie bag!

The Dessert Dilemma

In watching your total carbohydrate intake, you are continually learning how to incorporate foods you like into your meals. Dessert is no exception, but you can't afford to have your blood sugar skyrocket. If you carefully follow your meal plan or other eating program such as carbohydrate counting, you can eat a small portion of dessert.

You may want to avoid the desserts that are higher in sugar and fat. Try to find low-calorie, nonfat choices. A small portion of nonfat frozen yogurt in place of one bread exchange may be just the thing.

Alcohol

Alcoholic beverages often are served at restaurants and on social occasions, such as parties and holiday get-togethers. Many people with diabetes can drink alcohol—in moderation! But you first should consult with your doctor, because alcohol can interfere with the management of your diabetes or interact with other drugs you are taking. For more information on the effects of alcohol on diabetes, see Chapter 21.

Be Realistic

Accept the fact that nothing is perfect in life. Whether you are eating at home or away, do the best you can. Remember that meal plans are guidelines designed to give you flexibility—your meals are not set in stone.

Be ready for minor setbacks. If the waiter mistakenly douses your salad with dressing, politely send it back. If you initially have trouble converting exchanges or figuring out what the total amount of carbohydrate is in a meal at restaurants, don't despair. It will get easier with practice. And if you have a momentary lapse, realize that everyone slips once in a while. Just pick up where you left off and continue your diabetes management with a positive outlook.

Below are two lists of terms you'll often find on restaurant menus. When ordering, use these lists to help make wise decisions.

THUMBS UP!

The following words describe ingredients or preparation styles that are relatively low in fat, cholesterol, and calories compared with other items on the menu.

baked	barbecued
broiled	(watch sugar content)
boiled	marinated
charbroiled	kabob
steamed	sautéed in light wine sauce
roasted	light mushroom sauce
stir-fried	tomato-based sauce
(request unsaturated oil, such as	teriyaki sauce*
olive, corn, or canola oil)	Oriental sauce*
simmered	lemon sauce
stewed	on bed of mixed vegetables
poached	with herbs and spices
grilled	cooked with curry
(often done to fish)	Cajun style
mesquite-grilled	low-calorie dressing
blackened	

* High-sodium.

THUMBS DOWN!

Watch out for these words on menus. These ingredients or preparation styles are usually higher in fat, cholesterol, and calories.

fried	Newburg
deep-fried	Thermidor
pan-fried	à la mode
breaded and fried	butter
batter-fried	sour cream
crispy	duck
stuffed	bacon
au gratin	sausage
served with gravy	cheese (grated, melted)
rich sweet sauce	blue cheese
creamy	hollandaise
creamy wine sauce	mayonnaise
creamy cheese sauce	guacamole
sweet-sour sauce	crisp tortilla
en casserole	coconut milk

Lists adapted from: *The Restaurant Companion: A Guide to Healthier Eating Out* (Hope Warshaw, Chicago: Surrey Books, 1990).

Fast-Food Choices

Fast-food restaurants offer convenient, quick meals at reasonable prices. However, they also are known for high-fat, high-calorie foods. In fact, it is easy to consume five or more "fat choices" in one meal. By planning ahead, you can save your daily fat choices for an occasional fast-food meal. The Food Choice Lists in the Appendix can help you incorporate fast-food selections into your meal plan.

Better yet, order something lower in fat. Some fast-food restaurants are offering leaner selections such as skim milk, baked potato, or lettuce salads. Some are even beginning to offer leaner burgers, made with protein fillers like seaweed and soybean curd (tofu). You can also order burgers that are grilled, not fried, and grilled chicken sandwiches. However, be aware that many items that fast-food restaurants call low-fat may not be low enough in fat for you to eat very often.

Ethnic Cuisine

Many international dishes will fit into your meal plan. Ask your dietitian about cuisines such as Italian, Chinese, Mexican, or Indian. Also, consider buying a book on ethnic foods (see book list on page 313).

Eating with family and friends is one of life's greatest pleasures. That doesn't have to change just because you have diabetes. You can enjoy a wide variety of delicious foods and still stick to your meal plan.

FIGURE 20-1. A SAMPLE MENU

Luncheon Menu

Usually smaller portions.

Available Every Day of the Week 11:00–3:30

Avoid fried foods as they are higher in fat.

Don't be afraid to ask for items to be prepared without fat or with margarine.

Ask for dressings on the side.

SANDWICHES	
Fresh Shrimp Roll	6.95
Fresh Crabcake Sandwich	7.95
Grilled Burger	5.50
Grilled Cheeseburger	5.75
Grilled Bacon Cheeseburger	5.95
Grilled Chicken	6.95
BBQ Chicken Sandwich	6.95
Grilled Chicken, Bacon, Cheese	6.95
Fried Clam Roll	8.95
Fried Scallop Roll	8.95
Fried Fish Sandwich	6.50
with cheese	6.95
Fresh Crabmeat Salad Roll	8.95
Fresh Lobster Roll	10.95
Oriental Chicken Salad Roll	5.50

ENTREES	
Broiled Scrod	6.95
Broiled Lemon Sole	7.95
Broiled or Grilled Bluefish	6.95
Broiled Haddock	8.95
Grilled Seafood Sampler	8.95
BBQ Shrimp Kabob	8.95
Chicken Teriyaki	6.95
BBQ Chicken Breast	6.95
Fried Scrod	6.95
Fried Lemon Sole	7.95
Fried Calamari	6.50
Fish and Chips	6.50
Broiled or Grilled Catfish	7.50
Ginger Calamari	6.75
Broiled/Grilled Coho Salmon	8.95
Fried Haddock	8.95
Grilled Salmon Trout	7.95
Fresh Sunshine Tilapia	6.95

SALADS	
Jumbo Shrimp	*8.95
Calamari Pasta Vinaigrette	*6.95
Seafood Emporium	*9.50
Shrimp and Curry	*7.95
Oriental Chicken Salad	*7.95
Fresh Maine Crabmeat	*9.25
Oriental Shrimp Salad	*7.95
Fresh Lobster Salad	*11.95
Fresh Garden Salad	*2.50
with chowder or soup	*4.95
Fresh Caesar Salad	*3.95
with chowder or soup	*5.95
Poached Salmon Salad	*8.95

All luncheon entrees and sandwiches are served with homebaked rolls, fresh country cole slaw and choice of French fries, baked potato, rice pilaf or sweet potato chips, except where "*" appears

Ask the waiter to remove the bread basket if it is too much temptation. Substitute a salad or a vegetable dish.

FIGURE 20-2. MEAL-PLAN CARD

BREAKFAST
Number of Choices   Time _____
_____ Milk
_____ Fruit
_____ Bread/Starch
_____ Meat
_____ Fat

MORNING SNACK   Time _____

LUNCH
Number of Choices   Time _____
_____ Milk
_____ Fruit
_____ Vegetable
_____ Bread/Starch
_____ Meat
_____ Fat

AFTERNOON SNACK   Time _____

DINNER
Number of Choices   Time _____
_____ Milk
_____ Fruit
_____ Vegetable
_____ Bread/Starch
_____ Meat
_____ Fat

EVENING SNACK   Time _____

CHAPTER 21

Alcohol, Drugs, and Diabetes

PEOPLE WITH DIABETES don't live in a vacuum. Just like everyone else, they get cold viruses, headaches, and other medical problems that need to be treated with drugs, either over-the-counter medications or prescription drugs. Overall, people with diabetes can take almost any medication that people without diabetes use. But you need to be wary of possible problems. In general, the best advice is to always check with your doctor.

In addition to over-the-counter medications and prescription drugs, there are the so-called recreational drugs—both legal and illegal. Two of the most commonly used legal recreational drugs in the United States are *alcohol*, found in beverages, and *nicotine*, a component of tobacco. Illegal drugs include *marijuana*, *cocaine*, and *heroin*. These drugs can have a considerable impact on your diabetes management.

All drugs are chemicals that your body must handle—at the same time it is handling your diabetes and converting food into energy. That's why you should be aware of how such drugs may interact with your diabetes.

OVER-THE-COUNTER MEDICATIONS

You can probably use most of the over-the-counter drugs used by people who don't have diabetes. However, there are some exceptions. For example, you should be cautious with medicines that are highly sweetened, such as cough remedies that use concentrated syrups for a base. Occasionally, your doctor may allow you to use such medications, as long as you compensate for the increase in sugar.

You may be concerned about the information you read on the labels of over-the-counter medications such as decongestants or antihistamines. Many of these cold medications often state "not to be used in cases of hypertension, diabetes . . ." These medicines may stimulate the adrenal glands to produce adrenaline, which can raise blood sugar levels—but only slightly, if at all. These warnings exist primarily for legal reasons, to release the manufacturer from responsibility, although any actual risk for someone with diabetes is quite small. You can often overlook the warning on over-the-counter medications—provided your physician has approved of their use.

The real concern for people with diabetes is that they will use these medications to treat flu, not properly monitor for high blood sugar and ketones, and end up in diabetic ketoacidosis. Anyone with an illness such as flu should follow the sick-day rules (Chapter 13) and contact your health-care provider as needed.

Prescription Drugs

Drugs that require regulation for their use are available only by prescription. These regulations are a barricade to protect you from taking drugs that could be harmful. The prescription "lifts" the barricade, once your doctor has decided it is safe for you to take the drug according to strict guidelines.

Some prescription drugs can affect your diabetes management. For example, fluid pills (diuretics), cortisone, birth control pills, and estrogen supplements can raise your blood sugar levels. Diabetes treatments used in combination with alcohol, salicylates (such as aspirin), and beta blockers (taken by some people with heart problems) may promote or mask the symptoms of low blood sugar. So as you can see, problems can arise when you are taking a variety of prescription drugs. The important thing is to discuss all drugs you are taking with your doctor.

ALCOHOL

Although alcohol is a substance that is legal to use in a responsible manner, it is, in fact, a drug. Perhaps you are someone who has routinely enjoyed having an occasional drink on social occasions. Now that you have diabetes, can you continue that practice?

Many people with diabetes are able to drink alcoholic beverages. But it should always be done in moderation. A consultation with your doctor would be advisable because alcohol may interact with other drugs you are taking. If your doctor approves, you should have no more than one or two "alcohol equivalents" a day, preferably spread out over 2 hours or more. An alcohol equivalent is

- 4-ounce glass of wine.
- 12-ounce light beer.
- a mixed drink containing 1½ ounces of "hard liquor," such as scotch, whiskey, or vodka. It should be mixed with sugar-free soda. Don't use regular soda, juice, or mixes like Tom Collins, which contain a lot of carbohydrate and calories.

Alcohol can lower the blood sugar, causing extremely low-blood-sugar reactions in people who use insulin as well as those who take diabetes pills. Alcohol is absorbed directly from the stomach into the bloodstream and carried to the liver, where it is broken down. While the liver is processing alcohol, its ability to release sugar is almost completely blocked. In essence, the liver is "distracted" from doing its regular job. This can cause your blood sugar to drop and result in a low-blood-sugar reaction—up to 36 hours after drinking!

That is why you should eat while drinking. Food in the stomach slows down the absorption of alcohol into the bloodstream and reduces the amount of alcohol reaching the liver at any one time. The liver can then perform its other functions better, while also processing the smaller amount of alcohol.

If you're trying to lose weight, remember that alcohol itself is not a "free" food. It is high in calories and may slow down your weight-loss efforts. For example, a 12-ounce light beer, 4 ounces of wine, or 1½ ounces of hard liquor are each about 100 calories. Alcohol also stimulates the appetite, which could affect your diet.

How should you account for these extra calories? Should they be considered an "exchange" in your meal plan? If you use insulin, it is not recommended that you exchange the calories obtained through alcohol for the calories obtained through food. However, if you do *not* use insulin, you should compensate for the calories in your alcoholic beverage by reducing the number of calories in your meal plan, particularly if you are trying to lose weight. To help you do this, use Table 21-1, which shows the equivalent food group for different types of alcohol. Notice, for example, the calories in a regular 12-ounce beer are equal to 1 bread/starch plus 1½ fat choices (if you use an exchange meal plan). The regular beer contains 14 grams of carbohydrate, if you are using carbohydrate counting.

Liquors such as sweet wines, liqueurs, and cordials contain large quantities of carbohydrate and should be avoided because they can raise your blood sugar too high.

Alcohol can exacerbate complications of diabetes. If you have nerve-related problems (*neuropathy*) from diabetes, alcohol may make the condition worse. Alcohol can also cause unpleasant reactions under certain conditions. For example, if you take a diabetes pill called Diabinese, you may experience facial flushing or headaches when drinking alcohol. The symptoms are harmless, but can be frightening. Fortunately, they are temporary and will disappear in time. But people using this medication have good reason to avoid alcohol.

There is an excellent nonalcoholic option—alcohol-free beer. This beverage is socially acceptable, contains no alcohol, and has fewer calories and carbohydrates than regular beer (see Table 21-1).

Guidelines for Using Alcohol

- Use alcohol only after consulting with your health-care team. Alcohol may interfere with the proper management of your diabetes. However, if it doesn't and you wish to drink, your doctor and dietitian can discuss how to include alcohol in your eating plan—in moderation!
- Use alcohol only when your diabetes is under good control.
- Limit alcohol consumption if you are trying to lose weight. It is high in calories and also tends to increase the appetite.
- Know which types of alcohol are best. Avoid sweet wines, liqueurs, and cordials. They contain large amounts of carbohydrate.
- Mix hard liquor such as gin, rum, whiskey, bourbon, scotch, and vodka with water or sugar-free mixers.
- Don't drink alcohol on an empty stomach. If drinking before your evening meal, use the appetizers as part of your meal.

TABLE 21-1. FITTING ALCOHOL INTO YOUR MEAL PLAN

The use of alcohol should be discussed with your physician. As a general guideline, for persons using insulin, two alcoholic beverages may be used in addition to their regular meal plan. No food should be omitted in exchange for an alcoholic drink. For persons not on insulin who are watching their weight, alcohol is best substituted for fat choices and in some cases extra bread/starch choices.

Some alcoholic beverages, such as sweet wines, sweet vermouth and wine coolers, contain higher amounts of sugar and carbohydrate. Use these sparingly as they may increase your blood sugar levels too much.

BEVERAGE	AMOUNT (OUNCES)	CALORIES	CARBOHY-DRATE (GRAMS)	EQUAL TO:
Beer				
Regular beer	12	150	14	1 bread/starch and 1½ fats
Light beer	12	100	6	2 fats
Nonalcoholic beer	11	50	10	1 bread/starch
Distilled spirits				
86 proof (gin, rum, vodka, whiskey, scotch, bourbon)	1.5	105	trace	2 fats
Wine				
Red table or rosé	4	85	1.0	2 fats
Dry white	4	80	.4	2 fats
Sweet wine	2	90	6.5	½ bread/starch and 1½ fats
Light wine	4	55	1.3	1 fat
Wine coolers	12	190	22.0	1½ fruit and 3 fat
Champagne	4	100	3.6	2 fats
Sherry	2	75	1.5	1½ fats
Sweet sherry/port	2	95	7.0	½ bread/starch and 1½ fats
Vermouths				
Dry	3	105	4.2	2 fats
Sweet	3	140	13.9	1 bread/starch and 2 fats

SMOKING AND NICOTINE

Smoking can affect people with diabetes in numerous ways—all of them harmful. Smoking belongs in a discussion of drugs primarily because of *nicotine*, the major chemical absorbed by the body from smoking. It causes the blood vessels to constrict, or become narrowed. People with diabetes are already at a higher risk for blood-vessel disease. Therefore, smoking adds an additional risk for such problems as heart disease and stroke.

Smoking is also the leading cause of cancer. It is, in fact, a great health hazard to modern society. It should be eliminated. If you have diabetes and smoke, the message couldn't be stronger: *Stop!*

What does it take to quit? A complete change in attitude. It won't do any good to say, "Well, I'll join a stop-smoking group and see how it goes." You must be ready to quit. You must be willing to make changes in your life. You must replace smoking with new and healthier habits. Once you reach this level of commitment, pick a "Quit Day." (Make it tomorrow!) Think of this day as taking charge of your life. Tell yourself, I don't have to smoke anymore. Then take the following actions:

- Hide the ashtrays. Throw away all cigarettes and lighters.
- Avoid caffeine and alcohol—they increase craving.
- Change your eating habits. Eat slowly. Leave the table right after eating and brush your teeth. You'll love the fresh taste!
- Spend time in nonsmoking areas—places usually not associated with smoking, such as the library.
- When the urge to smoke comes, do the "three Ds":

—*Delay:* Hold out for 3 minutes. The urge will pass.

—*Dampen the urge:* Do a mental sidestep, quietly telling yourself that this urge is not going to change your commitment.

—*Do something else:* Drink a glass of water. Take a walk. Take some deep breaths. Chat with a friend on the phone.

DRUG ABUSE AND MISUSE

The presence of illegal drugs in society is both a crime and a tragedy. Again, if you are using such drugs, stop! They are illegal for a purpose—they are dangerous to your health! Realizing that stopping is easier to say than to do, your first step should be *to resolve* to stop. Then talk to your health-care provider, who can help you find a program that will be successful.

If you are using drugs for so-called recreational purposes, you should realize the effect is just the opposite. Many illegal drugs are addictive and you will be unable to control their use. Instead, they will control you.

Apart from the wide range of problems that come with addiction, illegal drugs can also affect diabetes management. For example, high doses of *marijuana* can cause low blood sugar. In fact, marijuana may even hide low-blood-sugar reactions. It also causes people to eat frequently, which could result in high blood sugar. Moreover, many people who use marijuana for a long time say they develop a lack of interest in many aspects of life. Such apathy can have a negative impact on people with diabetes, who need to stick to a coordinated program of meal planning, medication, and monitoring.

What about drugs such as *heroin, cocaine,* and *morphine*? These drugs severely impair judgment, something that's critical to the proper care of diabetes. They can also increase blood sugar levels. Cocaine may decrease the appetite, which can disrupt a person's eating schedule. *Amphetamines,* commonly called "speed," can cause blood sugar to rise and also cause nervousness. Amphetamines are sometimes used by people as "diet pills" to help them lose weight. This strategy doesn't work, because most people gain back whatever they lost once they "get off" the diet pills.

In short, everyone—whether they have diabetes or not—should avoid the trap of using illegal drugs. The human costs are just too high.

What about drugs that are legal but can be misused? In large amounts, *caffeine* (commonly found in coffee, tea, and cola) can make your blood sugar rise. For this reason, people with diabetes should drink only a moderate amount of beverages containing caffeine. Also be wary of misusing medications such as tranquilizers and sleeping pills. Many people become dependent upon these drugs.

THE BEST MEDICINE

The body is a very complex system, with a countless number of chemical reactions going on at all times. The chemistry of a new drug can throw your body completely out of balance. You will benefit from doing everything you can to keep the chemistry of your body as normal as possible. If you use any type of drug, be sure to check with your physician. This policy is the best medicine yet!

CHAPTER 22

Traveling with Diabetes

For many people, traveling is one of the delights of their lives. They find the sights and sounds of new places, along with a break in normal routines, quite refreshing. They enjoy visiting friends and relatives in other parts of the country or traveling to foreign countries. You don't need to hesitate taking a camping trip, visiting friends, or even taking an around-the-world cruise just because you have diabetes. With adequate planning, you can care for your diabetes while traveling just as well as you manage at home.

PLANNING FOR TRAVEL

It's best to plan your travel as far ahead as possible. Once you know your destination, how you are traveling there, and how long you'll be staying, you can make the following preparations.

A Medical Checkup

Visit your doctor to be sure that your general health is okay and that your diabetes is in good control. Ask your doctor to write a letter on letterhead stationery explaining in detail your condition and any complications that another physician would need to know to take proper care of you. The letter may also come in handy in case you are ever questioned about the medications, syringes, and other medical items you are carrying. You will want to ask your doctor about medications to combat motion sickness or diarrhea. Such problems can be very disruptive to your diabetes management.

Immunizations

If you are traveling to areas of the world where immunizations are required, get them at least 1 month before your departure date. That way, your doctor will have plenty of time to deal with any effect they may have on your diabetes control. Many international airports and public health departments have phone-in lines to provide up-to-date information on necessary immunizations for various parts of the world.

Extra Medications, Syringes, and Prescriptions

Plan to take extra supplies of diabetes pills, insulin, syringes, and any other medications you may need. Take twice as much as you expect to use during your trip. Also carry prescriptions for these medications, which you may need to fill if your supplies are misplaced. Ask your doctor to write the generic names of these drugs, because brand names may vary from country to country. For example, instead of Micronase, your prescription should state the generic name *glyburide*.

If the insulin you normally use isn't available in the area you plan to visit, your doctor can provide you with a prescription for an alternative form. Don't be alarmed if you encounter your form of insulin under a name you don't recognize. Also be prepared to find it in concentrations of U-40 and U-80, rather than U-100. To measure these dosages properly, you'll need a U-40 or U-80 syringe. Such adjustments are necessary only if you lose your supplies or are planning to stay in another country for an extended period of time. For most trips, you will be able to carry all the supplies that you regularly use at home.

Time Zones

If you are traveling across time zones, consult with your health-care team before leaving. They can help you schedule your medications, a topic discussed in greater detail later in this chapter. When scheduling air travel, try to fly during daylight hours to minimize disruption to your schedule.

Contacting Doctors

Your doctor may be able to provide you with the name of a doctor who practices in the area you're planning to visit. Or consult with your local or national office of the American Diabetes Association (see listing in

Chapter 24), which can put you in touch with people at affiliates along your travel route. They can also provide you with names of physicians in those areas.

If traveling in foreign countries, ask the International Diabetes Federation (see Chapter 24) for the names of diabetes associations, which will know diabetes specialists in the countries you are visiting. Once you arrive, American embassies and consulates will be at your service, and your hotels may also keep a roster of English-speaking doctors. In an emergency, you should go to the nearest hospital.

Identification

Prepare to carry a form of identification in your purse or billfold that indicates you have diabetes (see Figure 22-1). This card also should contain your name, address, phone number, doctor's name and phone number, and the type and dose of insulin and other medications you use. Also wear a medical ID tag—a necklace or bracelet—that includes the name of your condition (diabetes) and an emergency phone num-

Figure 22-1

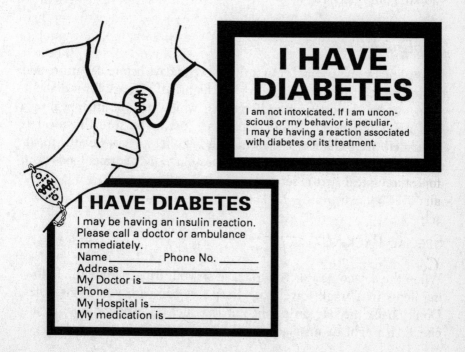

I HAVE DIABETES

I am not intoxicated. If I am unconscious or my behavior is peculiar, I may be having a reaction associated with diabetes or its treatment.

I HAVE DIABETES

I may be having an insulin reaction. Please call a doctor or ambulance immediately.

Name _____ Phone No. _____
Address _____
My Doctor is _____
Phone _____
My Hospital is _____
My medication is _____

ber (see Figure 22-2). This will help other people know how to assist you in an emergency.

Figure 22-2

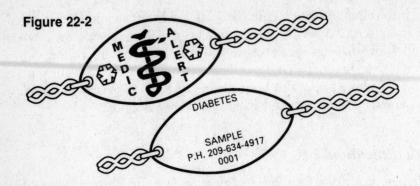

Before Departure

Before departure, find out if your health-insurance policy will cover you throughout your trip. Carry your health-insurance identification card. If traveling to a foreign country, learn how to say, "I have diabetes," "Please give me orange juice or sugar," and "Please get me a doctor" in the appropriate language. You may want to have these comments in writing in your wallet in the native language of the place you are going, as well.

Airplane Meals

If traveling by air, contact your airline several days before departure and ask for a "heart-healthy" meal for the flight. (If you ask for a diabetic meal, it often is just fruit and crackers, which may be unappealing.) Call again three days before departure, just to be sure the meal is scheduled. If by chance, the airline doesn't offer a heart-healthy meal, don't be concerned. You usually will be able to pick correct foods from almost any meal that is served.

SPECIAL PACKING

When the day comes for you to leave on your trip, include the following items in a small travel bag. Keep this bag with you at all times. Don't check the bag on public carriers such as buses, trains, or airplanes. It might be misplaced.

Carry-On Bag

- *Insulin.* Include all the insulin you will need for your entire trip. Watch out for temperature extremes. Insulin does not need to be refrigerated, and it should not be exposed to temperatures below 35° F. The bottle you have opened and are using is good for 1 month if unrefrigerated, and for 3 months if kept in a refrigerator. All unopened bottles are good until the manufacturer's expiration date. Don't put insulin in a bag that will be stored in the luggage compartment of an airplane, because high-altitude temperatures may cause it to freeze. Also, insulin should not be exposed to temperatures above 90° F for any length of time. There are specific products you may buy to keep diabetes supplies cool and safe while traveling. No ice is necessary with these products. Simply wrap a tissue around the bottle so it won't move around, put the lid on, and don't worry about it. If you use an insulin pump, bring extra batteries and supplies for the pump. Have a bottle of regular (short-acting) insulin and syringes with you for emergencies, even if you don't normally use this form of insulin. Also, take your glucagon kit, and instruct a companion how to use this medication in emergencies (see pages 177–178).
- *Diabetes Pills.* If your diabetes is treated with pills, be sure you pack these in your carry-on-bag.
- *Syringes.* Take all the syringes you will need during your trip. Use disposable syringes and be sure to dispose of them safely. Don't forget alcohol and cotton to use in wiping off the top of the insulin bottle and the injection site.
- *Monitoring Supplies.* Include all your supplies for blood sugar monitoring. If you use a glucose meter, take extra batteries and glucose strips that can be read as a back-up. Don't forget supplies to test for ketones.
- *Snacks.* Prepare a snack-pack containing carbohydrates to eat in case of low blood sugar (see list on page 172). Travel often involves unexpected delays in your meal schedule, so always carry some carbohydrate and protein foods, such as fruit, crackers, cheese, and peanut butter sandwiches. If you use some of your food supplies, replenish them at your first opportunity.

Traveling often involves considerable walking. So always pack an extra pair of comfortable shoes in your suitcase. Don't forget to take a mild antiseptic, moisture-restoring cream, foot powders, and emery boards for proper nail care.

ON THE WAY

Don't Skip Meals or Snacks

If traveling by car, be prepared to eat carbohydrate and protein foods (noted above) when there are meal delays. Also keep carbohydrate-containing foods in your car in case of a low-blood-sugar reaction. If this happens while you are driving, pull off the road, treat the low blood sugar (see Chapter 12), and wait at least 10 to 15 minutes before resuming your drive. If you tend to have low blood sugar, you might want to eat a snack of one (1) bread choice every two hours.

Exercise

Exercise is important while traveling. If you're on an airplane or train for a long period of time, occasionally walk up and down the aisle to stimulate circulation. If on a bus trip, take advantage of stops by getting off and taking a short walk. If driving in a car, plan to stop and stretch your legs every 1½ hours or so.

Tell Your Companions

If you're traveling with relatives or friends, let them know about your diabetes. They can adapt their plans to meet your needs and can also be of assistance.

Adjust Medication for Time Zones

If you are crossing time zones, ask your doctor or nurse educator if you should modify your insulin dose or injection schedule. A coast-to-coast trip within the United States means only a 3-hour time difference, something that usually requires minimal adjustment. But for longer trips with a time change of several hours, such as a trip to Europe, you may be advised to increase or decrease the amount of insulin in proportion to the time you will gain or lose. Check with your health-care team before leaving.

If you take more than one injection, think of your travel day as being lengthened or shortened at the end. While your first dose will probably go unchanged, the later ones will be either increased or decreased. If you need an in-flight injection, put half as much air into the insulin bottle as you normally would. This will compensate for the lower cabin pressure at high altitudes. If you take diabetes pills, you probably won't need to adjust your doses for time changes, particularly if you use a long-acting form.

Once you arrive at your destination, switch to the local time. When you wake up in the morning, resume your normal schedule of meals, exercise, and medication. Beware of jet lag, a fatigue that sometimes occurs with long-distance air travel. Be sure to give yourself a rest.

Sampling Local Foods

Throughout your trip, monitor your blood sugar levels frequently. In the beginning, your readings probably won't be normal because of all the excitement and change from your usual routine. Once you've brought your blood sugar to normal readings, you can sample local dishes freely. But don't go overboard—you don't have to eat every snack and beverage offered. As always, go easy on the alcohol.

Become familiar with the calories, carbohydrate and fat content of different foods. If you're not sure of a dish's ingredients, be sure to ask. When experimenting with new foods, be sure to monitor your blood sugar, preferably before eating and 2 hours after a meal.

Prevent Diarrhea and Motion Sickness

Diarrhea is an unpleasant problem for anyone. But for people with diabetes, it is especially dangerous because it can deplete the body of fluids and unabsorbed nutrients, upsetting the balance between your insulin dose and the sugar left in your system. To prevent "traveler's diarrhea" while on your trip, be wary of peeled fruits, leafy vegetables, undercooked meats, and milk products like cheese and cream sauces, especially in South and Central America, Asia, and Africa. These foods may contain bacteria that cause intestinal upset. Also avoid tap water and ice cubes. Instead, drink bottled water and tea, which usually are safe because the water has been boiled.

Motion sickness also can disrupt your normal eating schedule and fluid balance. Your health-care team can suggest medication to help prevent this problem.

CHAPTER 23

Especially for Family and Friends

IF YOU ARE CLOSE TO someone with diabetes—a family member or a friend—you are in a unique position. Indeed, you may not have diabetes yourself. But you will need to know quite a lot about diabetes and its treatment. In fact, the more you know, the easier life will be for the person with diabetes and the entire family. If you are a baby-sitter or caregiver who is temporarily taking care of a child with diabetes, you also need to have a basic understanding of diabetes and its treatment, and what to do in an emergency.

Why does the whole family have to get involved? First of all, diabetes is a *chronic* disorder—it will never go away. Unlike taking an antibiotic to rid the body of an infection, there is no magic wand to cure diabetes. It is something your loved one will have to deal with for life. Simply by virtue of living with this person, you cannot help but get involved.

Second, diabetes is something that requires a lot of *self-care*. In other words, people with diabetes themselves have to do most of the things necessary to take care of their disorder. They simply can't go to a doctor for a "quick" fix. And in caring for their health, people with diabetes need the help of family members—perhaps support for trying new treatments, or encouragement when things aren't going right.

Third, diabetes treatment requires constant *commitment*. Controlling diabetes takes a good deal of time and attention to daily routine. Your friend or loved one can never put diabetes on the "back burner." It will always be present and must be dealt with in a constructive manner. So, for friends and family members, it is important to have a working knowledge of diabetes and its care. With this knowledge, you can truly "be there" for the person with diabetes. You can help in everyday situations and during emergencies. And you will understand the coping skills that you, too, will need to deal with diabetes.

This chapter is for anyone who knows someone with diabetes. If you have diabetes and want a friend, co-worker, or family members to understand it better, give them this chapter to read. It can be the beginning of better understanding.

WHAT IS DIABETES?

Diabetes is a disruption in the way the body uses food for energy. It does not come from eating too much sugar. It relates to the way the body uses a form of sugar called *glucose*, which is absorbed into the bloodstream from the foods you eat. If not used properly, the sugar in your blood can rise too high, possibly causing a medical emergency.

The problem centers around the way the body produces and uses a substance called *insulin*. Think of insulin as the chemical "key" that unlocks the cells. It lets the sugar (glucose) that is circulating in your bloodstream into your body's cells. Everyone needs insulin. Without it, you can't survive. Insulin is made by the body in an organ called the pancreas. In people who don't have diabetes, this happens automatically. When you eat, the pancreas responds by making more insulin.

Type I Diabetes

In this form of diabetes, the pancreas has somehow been damaged and it can no longer produce insulin. People with Type I diabetes must get insulin from an outside source—through an injection (a "shot"). Insulin can't be taken by mouth because the stomach juices would destroy it. People who *depend* on injected insulin have Type I diabetes, also called *insulin-dependent diabetes*. This is the form of diabetes that often strikes before age 30.

Symptoms of Type I diabetes include

· Frequent urination
· Increased thirst
· Extreme hunger

- Unexplained weight loss
- Extreme fatigue
- Blurred vision

Type II Diabetes

Another form of diabetes is called *non-insulin-dependent diabetes* or Type II diabetes. This is the most common form of the disorder and often occurs in people after age 40. In this type of diabetes, the pancreas can still produce some insulin. But the insulin is ineffective (a condition called "insulin resistance" because the body "resists" the effects of insulin.) They may also produce too little insulin to overcome this resistance. People with Type II diabetes don't have to get their insulin from an outside source to survive. But to help boost the effectiveness of their own insulin, they may take oral medications, commonly called "diabetes pills." Sometimes, however, they do need to use insulin injections to supplement their own supply.

Symptoms of Type II diabetes include

- Any Type I symptom (listed above)
- Tingling or numbness in the hands or feet
- Frequent skin or vaginal infections

How Is Diabetes Treated?

Diabetes is never cured. It's just *managed*. In other words, the person who has diabetes must do a number of things to keep his or her blood sugar in control. This is true for both Type I and Type II diabetes. The treatment of diabetes is much like a balancing act. There are three main parts to this act—meal planning, exercise, and medication. In addition, people with diabetes must regularly perform tests on their blood to be sure that their blood sugar levels are under control. They are trying to keep them within the normal range of 60–140 mg/dl.

Meal Planning

This is an eating strategy, based on the individual needs of the person with diabetes. Designed with the help of a *registered dietitian*, the meal plan takes into account how many calories a person needs to maintain a proper weight (or to lose weight, because being overweight can increase the body's resistance to insulin). A meal plan also provides good nutrition, balancing six main food groups, which are called "choices"—*milk, fruit, vegetable, bread, meat,* and *fat.* In addition to a balanced diet, people with diabetes should limit their intake of fat, sodium (salt), and cholesterol. While it was long thought that people with diabetes couldn't eat food with sugar in it, recently the American Diabetes Association concluded that it is the total amount of carbohydrate that someone eats which will influence their blood sugars. Sugary foods contain higher amounts of carbohydrates, so people with diabetes do need to watch how much they eat . . . but they can eat modest amounts of sugar-containing foods, with proper planning. People with diabetes should also use alcohol only occasionally, if at all, and only after getting permission from their doctor. To review meal planning and nutrition in the treatment of diabetes, see Chapters 3 and 4.

Exercise

Regular exercise plays an important role in diabetes. Exercise makes the body's cells more sensitive to insulin, which makes it more effective, allowing people with Type I diabetes to use less insulin. It also reduces the insulin resistance commonly found in Type II diabetes. In addition, exercise lowers the "bad" form of cholesterol and triglycerides in the blood, which can promote the buildup of fatty deposits in your blood vessels and lead to heart disease or stroke. For more on the benefits of exercise in the treatment of diabetes, see Chapter 5.

Medication

People with Type I diabetes need to take insulin injections, and the timing of these injections is related to when they eat and when they exercise. There are many forms of insulin, and they have different times when they are active. Some are fast, some are intermediate, and some take longer to act. The idea is to match the peak activity of the insulin with the time that glucose is in the bloodstream (see Chapter 8). Some people with Type II diabetes take "diabetes pills," which boost the production of natural insulin in their bodies (see Chapter 7). These, too, are timed with meals and exercise.

Monitoring

People with diabetes must frequently test their blood sugar. That's because their pancreas is no longer on "automatic," and to compensate, they must determine the level of their blood sugar and make the correct response. They must also test for ketones, a sign that the body has turned to burning fat for fuel, which can lead to a dangerous condition called *ketoacidosis*. For more information on monitoring in the treatment of diabetes, see Chapter 10.

COMPLICATIONS FROM DIABETES

People who have diabetes are at risk for complications, which include problems with the eyes, kidneys, nerves, and other systems in the body. However, there is new evidence that by keeping their blood sugar in control as much as possible, people with diabetes can help reduce the chance that they will develop complications (see Chapter 17). Changes in the body's blood vessels are at the root of most of these complications. Frequent checkups at the doctor are important to detect and treat these problems before they become serious.

Eyes

Diabetic eye disease, called *retinopathy*, is caused by damage to the tiny blood vessels in the *retina*, the light-sensitive lining located in the back of the eye. If not treated, this damage can lead to problems with vision and even blindness. People with diabetes should have their eyes checked regularly (at least once a year) by an eye doctor, an *ophthalmologist*. If necessary, retinopathy can be treated with laser surgery.

Kidneys

Diabetes can damage the kidneys' ability to filter wastes from the blood, a complication called *nephropathy*. To prevent kidney damage, people with diabetes should keep their blood sugar in control. They should also do all they can to avoid developing high blood pressure (and have it treated if it develops). High blood pressure puts further strain on the kidneys. They also need to have their physician perform certain tests on a regular basis to identify kidney problems as early as possible.

Nerves

High blood sugar also can damage the nervous system, a condition called *neuropathy*. The result may be a coldness, tingling, or even unbearable pain in the legs or arms. Nerve damage can also upset other systems in the body, such as the digestive system. Medications can be prescribed that in some cases help ease these problems, and a person can also slow painful neuropathy by getting their blood sugar under better control.

Impotence

In men, nerve or blood-vessel damage can lead to *impotence*, the inability to achieve or maintain an erection. There are various ways to help treat this problem, including a device called a penile prosthesis, which is surgically inserted.

Blood Vessels

People with diabetes are more likely to develop blood-vessel disease than those who don't have diabetes. In general, the problem centers around a gradual thickening of the blood vessels, leading to either partial or total blockage, which may cause serious problems such as a heart attack or stroke. To help prevent blood-vessel disease, people with diabetes should eat a low-fat diet and get plenty of exercise. They should also reduce their blood pressure and not smoke!

Feet and Skin

People who have diabetes tend to have poorer blood circulation, which can impair the healing of skin. Sores or cuts can become a major problem, leading to infection. Nerve damage can make the problem even worse because the person may not notice the injury. Infections may occur, leading to gangrene and even amputation. To help avoid skin infections, people with diabetes should practice good foot care: inspect and bathe their feet daily, change socks frequently, and wear protective and comfortable shoes.

HOW TO DEAL WITH EMERGENCIES

People with diabetes can run into immediate trouble in two basic ways—when their blood sugar is too high, and when it is too low. Following are ways you can help in an emergency.

Insulin Reaction

Also called *hypoglycemia*, an insulin reaction occurs when blood sugar is too low. This can come on suddenly. *Symptoms*: sweating, shakiness, weakness, dizziness, nervousness, hunger, rapid heartbeat, irritability, confusion, and headache. Without treatment, the person can lose consciousness (sometimes called "insulin shock"). *What to do*: Give the person a sweet snack, such as hard candy or fruit juice (see list on page 172). If the person loses consciousness, give an injection of *glucagon*, a hormone that raises blood sugar (see pages 177–178 for instructions).

Ketoacidosis

Usually a complication of Type I diabetes, ketoacidosis generally doesn't happen suddenly. It is caused when blood sugar is so high that the body turns to fat stores for energy, leading to the production of ketones. Allowed to go untreated, this condition is life-threatening. *Symptoms*: nausea, stomach pain, vomiting, chest pain, rapid shallow breathing, difficulty staying awake. *What to do*: The person needs immediate emergency care. Call an ambulance. *Prevention*: By carefully monitoring blood sugar levels and urine ketone levels, particularly when ill, the person can take additional insulin to prevent ketoacidosis.

Hyperosmolar-Nonketotic Coma

Usually a complication of Type II diabetes, this condition occurs when blood sugar gets so high that the body becomes dehydrated, leading to a severe imbalance in the body's chemistry and convulsions. *Symptoms*: excessive thirst or urination, increased hunger, drowsiness, nausea or vomiting, abdominal pain, rapid shallow breathing. *What to do*: The person needs immediate emergency care. Call an ambulance. *Prevention*: Careful monitoring of blood sugar levels can alert the person, particularly when ill, to rising blood sugar so advice can be sought from the health-care team before hyperosmolar-nonketotic coma occurs.

YOUR SUPPORT AND ENCOURAGEMENT

As a family member or friend, you can play a key role in the care of someone with diabetes. If you are a parent of a child with diabetes, you initially will be very much involved (see Chapter 14). But by the time your child nears adulthood, it's best if you have slowly transferred all of these duties, allowing your child to manage as independently as possible. That's because people with diabetes can best manage their care if they are self-reliant. In other words, they achieve the most success when they understand and fully accept the responsibility of their treatment program—meal plan, exercise, medication schedule, and self-testing of blood sugar.

As a friend or family member, however, you don't need to stay completely out of the picture. People with diabetes need a lot of encouragement and support. They are dealing with a very irksome and time-consuming problem. They sometimes can become depressed, upset, or frustrated (see Chapter 19). They can have "bad" days, in which they let their treatment slide. How should you react? Nagging is not the answer. Instead, it's more helpful to ask if there's anything you can do to help. Or ask if anything is bothering them, perhaps something apart from diabetes. The everyday stresses of life can take a toll on anyone, and in people with diabetes such problems can seem even heavier. In essence, make yourself available to listen and help.

If you're in charge of meals, you're already providing a valuable service. But try to resist making the food choices for a person with diabetes. As for your role in the exercise program, it may work out fine for you to participate—we all need regular exercise! But remember, it's important for every person with diabetes to develop a routine that he or she can maintain independently. Your friend or family member shouldn't rely too much on your participation. And finally, if you are considering getting married to someone with diabetes, there are issues that you and your prospective spouse need to sort out. For special guidance in this area, read Chapters 15 and 16.

You can be a valuable partner in helping someone with diabetes. But be aware that diabetes can dramatically change the dynamics of a family. It can cause stress in even the most stable relationships. In fact, there may be times that *you* need support and encouragement. Don't forget to take care of your own physical and emotional needs. Don't hesitate to seek the guidance of a professional counselor. Such an approach will do a world of good for you—and for the person you are trying to help.

Roles, Rights, and Resources

MANY PEOPLE WILL BE involved in caring for your diabetes—you and your health-care team, and perhaps members of your family or a special friend. You should know how to select the doctor who will oversee your care, as well as the other professionals on your health-care team and the services they can provide. You should also be aware of your rights as a person with diabetes and take advantage of other resources that you and your family can use to find out more about diabetes.

ROLES OF YOUR HEALTH-CARE TEAM

Today's world of medicine is very specialized. In caring for your diabetes, it is likely that your medical needs will be met by a number of health-care professionals. If at all possible, you should find a medical setting where your diabetes is cared for by a team of professionals, each an expert in a particular aspect of your total care. The team should include:

- *Primary-care physician*—a physician who practices general medicine, often called a general practitioner, internist (certified in internal medicine), or family practitioner (certified in family medicine). This doctor is trained to care for the whole person and treat a wide range of medical problems, including illnesses other than diabetes, checking cholesterol levels, giving flu shots, doing screening tests for early signs of cancer, treating minor injuries, etc. Your primary-care physician is a very important part of your diabetes care. Although he or she may be treating other problems besides diabetes, you should be sure that this doctor is experienced and interested in the care of people with diabetes. A good primary-care physician will know his or her limitations and will refer you to specialists, such as a diabetologist or other members of the health-care team when needed.

- *Diabetologist*—a physician with specialized training in the management of diabetes. Alternatively, your diabetes care may be provided by an *endocrinologist*, a physician who cares for diabetes along with other diseases of glands and hormones. (Most endocrinologists are knowledgeable about diabetes, but some may focus their practice in caring for particular gland or bodily functions not directly associated with diabetes, such as hormones related to sexual function and reproduction). In either case, you want someone trained and experienced in diabetes care.

- *Diabetes nurse educator* (D.N.E.)—a nurse who provides the guidance and training that you will need in the day-to-day management of diabetes, answers questions about any problems you may be having with your diabetes, and helps you make the necessary changes in your lifestyle. This person may also be a certified diabetes educator (C.D.E.).

- *Registered dietitian* (R.D.)—a professional who assesses your nutritional needs and tailors the goals of your meal plan according to your food preferences, budget, and lifestyle. This person, too, may be a certified diabetes educator.

- *Exercise physiologist*—a professional who assesses your needs for physical activity and devises an exercise program to help you maintain optimal control of your diabetes. Your exercise specialist also may be a certified diabetes educator.

- *Ophthalmologist*—a physician trained in detecting and treating eye problems early to reduce your risk of diabetic eye disease.

- *Mental health professional*—a professional who is trained to counsel patients with a chronic disorder such as diabetes. The mental health expert is there to help you sort through and handle any emotional and social problems you may be having in living with diabetes.

SELECTING YOUR HEALTH-CARE TEAM

Choosing a health-care team may take some time but is well worth the effort. Such professionals are available at specialized centers, such as Joslin Diabetes Center in Boston and its affiliated centers in other parts of the country. They may also be found at medical centers affiliated with medical schools. In choosing your health-care team, you may want to ask a trusted doctor, nurse, or knowledgeable friend for recommendations. It is necessary to find a team of professionals with whom you feel comfortable and confident. Ultimately, the decision is yours. That's why it is very important that you know something about diabetes care. As a health-care consumer, you will be better able to recognize the right team when you find one.

Below is a list of criteria that reflects desirable qualities to seek in a diabetes health-care team. Use this list as a guide to help choose the team best for you.

- They are knowledgeable about diabetes and its care.
- They listen to your concerns and help you identify solutions to the problems.
- They are sensitive to the challenges of life with diabetes.
- They return phone calls within an appropriate time.
- They consult you and consider your lifestyle, likes, dislikes, and abilities when developing your diabetes-care program.
- They work with you to help maintain the best diabetes control possible.
- They help you learn as much as possible about diabetes and how to prevent complications.
- They routinely perform necessary tests and evaluations.
- In accordance with the findings of the Diabetes Control and Complications Trial, they believe it is very important to keep your blood sugar as close to normal as possible.
- They participate in activities of the American Diabetes Association.

YOUR ROLES AND RIGHTS

People with diabetes play a significant role in their care. Your diabetes team will consider your needs, concerns, and lifestyle when working with you to manage your diabetes. Nonetheless, you are the key person on the diabetes team. Your responsibility is to carry out the treatment program—that is, to be involved with the "self-care" of your diabetes. On a daily basis you will be responsible for monitoring your blood sugar, selecting your food choices, exercising, and taking medications. You will interpret your blood sugar levels and make informed decisions about how to daily fine-tune your care. But along with responsibility for care, you have the right to be informed about your diabetes and your risks for developing complications. This right also includes knowing what options are available to care for your diabetes and any complications, along with your overall health.

There is a lot to know and remember when caring for your diabetes. The list below will help you sort out what to do to ensure your diabetes is being treated at an optimal level. The American Diabetes Association, American Association of Diabetes Educators, and other groups are continually revising their recommendations for people with diabetes in light of new research results. The following list represents Joslin's and their thinking as this book was being developed.

Appointments

Consultation with members of your health-care team will vary with each individual, but should include at least the following number of visits:

Primary-care physician—at least once a year for general care; more frequently if specific problems arise

Diabetes specialist—2 times a year unless your physician recommends more frequent visits (the American Diabetes Association recommends people using insulin see their diabetes specialist every 3 months)

Nurse educator—you should receive educational training at least once a year, more frequently when you are newly diagnosed or changing your treatment program

Dietitian—at least once a year to update and revise your eating program; you may need more help when you are newly diagnosed or changing your treatment program

Exercise physiologist—at least once a year to review your fitness level and make any adjustments necessary for diabetes management

Ophthalmologist (eye doctor)—once a year; more often if problems arise

Mental health specialist
   —when diagnosed with diabetes-related health problems
   —when life with diabetes becomes disruptive to everyday life
   —during any life crisis

Self-Care Skills

People with diabetes should develop the following knowledge and skills important to self-care:

SELF-MONITORING OF BLOOD SUGAR
   —use of glucose monitor
   —keeping a record of times that tests are performed, of results, and of other factors that affect diabetes management
   —interpreting your blood sugar levels to make appropriate changes in your treatment program

USE OF MEDICATION
   —knowledge of diabetes pills (Type II diabetes)
   —knowledge of types and action of insulin (if using insulin)
   —how to inject insulin
   —site rotation for injection
   —keeping a record of injections
   —proper storage and refrigeration of insulin

KNOWLEDGE OF HIGH AND LOW BLOOD SUGAR
   —causes
   —symptoms
   —treatment
   —prevention

MEAL PLANNING
   —meal plan techniques
   —special foods and occasions
   —dining out
   —portion control
   —guidelines for low-fat and low-cholesterol eating
   —weight goals

EXERCISE
   —basic components of an exercise prescription (duration, intensity, frequency, timing)
   —preventing low blood sugar

—adjustments for exercise, including snacking and reducing insulin dose

FOOT CARE
—daily foot care
—emergency treatment
—preventing foot problems related to diabetes

SICK-DAY MANAGEMENT
—how to prevent life-threatening problems
—what to eat and drink
—monitoring and medication schedule

URINE TESTING FOR KETONES
—significance of ketones
—when to monitor
—how to interpret ketone results

Tests by Professionals

The following tests should be performed by health-care professionals:

FOR DIABETES MANAGEMENT
—blood glucose (each visit, in addition to daily monitoring at home)
—glycosylated hemoglobin (2–4 times per year)
—urine analysis (each visit)
—blood lipids, including cholesterol (HDL and LDL) and triglycerides (once yearly; more if abnormal)
—comparison of your glucose monitor with lab results for meter accuracy (each visit)

KIDNEY AND MINERAL TESTS
—urine testing for protein (each visit)
—urine testing for microalbuminuria (once yearly)
—blood testing for electrolytes, blood urea nitrogen (BUN), and creatinine (once yearly; more often if abnormal or if you are using medications that might affect their values)
—urine testing for creatinine clearance (once yearly; more often if abnormal)

GENERAL HEALTH CARE
—blood chemistries and blood counts (once yearly; more often if abnormal)
—blood pressure (each visit)

Guidelines for Office Visits

Proper care of your diabetes involves working closely with a team of diabetes professionals. Following are guidelines for each visit.

ROUTINE VISITS
—check your blood pressure
—review your blood sugar values; also test your glycosylated hemoglobin
—review and clarify your target blood glucose levels
—eye examination (look in your eyes)
—foot examination
—discuss other health problems
—revise your diabetes treatment program, as necessary, including meal plan, exercise, monitoring schedule, medications, and foot care

ANNUAL VISIT
—all of the above
—complete physical examination
—review of self-care skills: how to use insulin or other diabetes medications, monitoring technique, treatment of low blood sugar, sick-day care
—dilated eye exam by an ophthalmologist
—tests to measure your kidney function
—evaluation of your risk factors for complications of diabetes: smoking, cholesterol levels, weight, and blood pressure

QUESTIONS TO ASK YOUR HEALTH-CARE TEAM

How should I be treating my diabetes?
How is my diabetes control?
What is my blood sugar level?
What is my glycosylated hemoglobin (A_{1C}) level and what does it mean?

What are my cholesterol and triglyceride levels and what do they
  mean?
How should I monitor my diabetes?
What is my diabetes meal plan?
What is my exercise program?
What should my blood sugar goals be?

WAYS TO LEARN MORE ABOUT DIABETES

Classes and programs at diabetes centers
Books and pamphlets
Sessions with diabetes educators
Support groups

DIABETES ORGANIZATIONS AND SOCIETIES

General Diabetes Information

American Diabetes Association, 1660 Duke Street, P.O. Box 25757,
Alexandria, Virginia 22314. Phone: (703) 549-1500, or toll-free
(800) 232-3472.

American Dietetic Association, 430 N. Michigan Avenue, Chicago,
Illinois 60611. Phone: (800) 877-1600.

National Diabetes Information Clearinghouse, 805 15th Street,
N.W., Room 500, Washington, D.C. 20005.

International Diabetes Federation, International Association Center,
40 Washington Street, B-1050, Brussels, Belgium. Phone: 32-2/647
44 14.

Children

Juvenile Diabetes Foundation, 432 Park Avenue South, New York,
New York 10016-8013. Phone: (212) 889-7575. Other offices located in Chatswood, Australia; Willowdale and Ontario, Canada;
London, England; Athens, Greece; Tel Aviv, Israel; São Paulo, Bra-
zil; Santiago, Chile; Paris, France; Calcutta, India; and Rome, Italy.

Joslin Diabetes Center and Its Affiliates

Joslin Diabetes Center is an international leader in diabetes treatment, research, patient and professional education affiliated with Harvard Medical School. Founded in 1898 in Boston, Massachusetts, the center now also has affiliated diabetes centers treating patients around the country.

Headquarters Centers

Joslin Diabetes Center
One Joslin Place
Boston, Massachusetts 02115
(617) 732-2440

Joslin Diabetes Center at Framingham
161 Worcester Road
Framingham, Massachusetts 01701
(508) 620-9600

Joslin-Lahey Diabetes Center
1 Essex Center Drive
Peabody, Massachusetts 01960
(508) 977-6336

Joslin/Deaconess-Nashoba Hospital
200 Groton Road
Ayer, Massachusetts 01432
(508) 772-0200/Ext. 451

Joslin Diabetes Center in Falmouth
316 Gifford Street
Falmouth, Massachusetts 02540
(508) 548-1944

Affiliated Centers

Joslin Center for Diabetes
Saint Barnabas Medical Center
101 Old Short Hills Road
West Orange, New Jersey 07052
(201) 325-6555

Joslin Center for Diabetes
Saint Barnabas, Community Medical Center Division
368 Lakehurst Road, Suite 305
Toms River, New Jersey 08753
(908) 349-5757

Joslin Center for Diabetes
Saint Barnabas, Princeton Division
100 Canal Pointe Blvd., Suite 100
Princeton, New Jersey 08540
(609) 987-0037

Joslin Center for Diabetes
Thomas Jefferson University Hospital/Wills Eye Hospital
211 South 9th Street, Suite 600
Philadelphia, Pennsylvania 19107
(215) 928-3400

Joslin Center for Diabetes
Western Pennsylvania Hospital
5140 Liberty Avenue
Pittsburgh, Pennsylvania 15224
(412) 578-1724

Nalle Clinic Diabetes Center, an affiliate of Joslin
1350 South Kings Drive
Charlotte, North Carolina 28207
(704) 342-8000

Joslin Center for Diabetes
Morton Plant Hospital
323 Jeffords Street
Clearwater, Florida 34616
(813) 461-8300

Joslin Center for Diabetes
Baptist Hospital of Miami
8900 North Kendall Drive
Miami, Florida 33176-2197
(800) 992-1879
(305) 270-3696

Joslin Center for Diabetes
Methodist Hospital of Indiana
1701 North Senate Boulevard

Box 1367
Indianapolis, Indiana 46206
(317) 929-8489

Joslin Center for Diabetes
MacNeal Medical Center
7020 West 79th Street
Bridgeview, Illinois 60455
(708) 430-0730

Joslin Center for Diabetes
St. Luke's–Roosevelt Hospital Center
425 West 59th Street
New York, New York 10019
(212) 523-8353

Opening soon:
Joslin Center for Diabetes
Straub Clinic and Hospital
Honolulu, Hawaii

Joslin Center for Diabetes
SUNY/Syracuse
Syracuse, New York 13210

JOSLIN BOOKS AND RESOURCES

Joslin offers a number of patient information and educational materials.
All of these publications are available directly from Joslin. For current
prices and purchasing information, contact Joslin Diabetes Center,
Publications Office, One Joslin Place, Boston, Massachusetts 02115;
phone (617) 732-2695; fax (617) 732-2562.

COOKBOOK

The Joslin Diabetes Gourmet Cookbook (Bonnie Polin, Fran Giedt,
and Joslin Nutrition Services Department, New York: Bantam
Books, 1994)

GUIDES, MANUALS, AND BOOKLETS FOR EVERYONE WITH DIABETES

Joslin Diabetes Manual, 12th ed. (Leo Krall and Richard Beaser,
Philadelphia: Lea & Febiger, 1989)
Good Health with Diabetes . . . through Exercise (1992)

Fighting Longterm Complications (1992)
Menu Planning—Simple! (1992)
Eating Well, Living Better (1992)
Weight Loss—A Winning Battle (1992)
The Foot Book (1992)

FOR INSULIN USERS

The Basics Pak for Insulin Users (1994)
Diabetes Treated with Insulin: A Short Guide (1994)
Diabetes Teaching Guide for People Who Use Insulin (1989)
Outsmarting Diabetes (R. Beaser, Minneapolis: Chronimed, 1994)

FOR NONINSULIN USERS

Type II Two-Pack (1992)
Managing Your Diabetes without Insulin (1992)

FOR CHILDREN

A Guide for Parents of Children and Youth with Diabetes (1987)
Everyone Likes to Eat, 2nd ed. (H. Holleroth et al., Minneapolis: Chronimed, 1993)

FOR SPECIAL POPULATIONS

A Guide for Women with Diabetes Who Are Pregnant . . . or Plan to Be (1987)

FOR PHYSICIANS

Joslin's Diabetes Mellitus, 13th ed. (C. Ronald Kahn and Gordon Weir, eds., Baltimore: Williams & Wilkins, 1994)

VIDEOS

Know Your Diabetes, Know Yourself (1987)
Living with Diabetes: A Winning Formula (1992)

OTHER BOOKS AND RESOURCES

COOKBOOKS

American Diabetes Association Holiday Cookbook (Betty Wedman, New York: Prentice-Hall, 1986)

American Diabetes Association Month of Meals, A Menu Planner (American Diabetes Association, 1660 Duke Street, Alexandria, Virginia 22314, 1989)

American Diabetes Association Special Celebrations and Parties Cookbook (Betty Wedman, New York: Prentice-Hall, 1989)

Creative Cooking for Renal Diabetic Diets (The Cleveland Clinic Foundation, Senay Publishing Inc., P.O. Box 397, Chesterland, Ohio 44026)

Diabetic Breakfast and Brunch Cookbook (Mary Jane Finsand, New York: Sterling Publishing, 1987)

Family Cookbook, vols. I, II, III, and IV (American Diabetes Association and American Dietetic Association, 1660 Duke Street, Alexandria, Virginia 22314)

The Guiltless Gourmet (Judy Gilliard and Joy Kirkpatrick, Nutrition Wise Partnership, P.O. Box 499, Rancho Mirage, California, 1990)

The Guiltless Gourmet Goes Ethnic (Judy Gilliard and Joy Kirkpatrick, Minneapolis: DCI Publishing, 1990)

The High Fiber Cookbook for Diabetics (Mabel Cavaiani, New York: Perigee Books, 1987)

Jane Brody's Good Food Book (Jane Brody, New York: W.W. Norton, 1985)

Jane Brody's Good Food Gourmet (Jane Brody, New York: W.W. Norton, 1990)

The Joy of Snacks (Nancy Cooper, Diabetes Center, Inc., 2851 Hedberg Drive, Minnetonka, Minnesota 55343)

The Living Heart Diet (Michael DeBakey, New York: Raven Press/ Simon & Schuster, 1984)

The Restaurant Companion: A Guide to Healthier Eating Out (Hope Warshaw, Chicago: Surrey Books, 1990)

FOOD EXCHANGES

Convenience Food Facts (Arlene Monk and Marion Franz, International Diabetes Center, Park Nicollet Medical Foundation, 4959 Excelsior Boulevard, Minneapolis, Minnesota 55416)

The Diabetic's Brand Name Food Exchange Handbook (Andrea Barrett, Philadelphia: Running Press)

Exchanges for All Occasions (Marion Franz, International Diabetes Center, Park Nicollet Medical Foundation, 4959 Excelsior Boulevard, Minneapolis, Minnesota 55416)

FAT-GRAM COUNTING

The Fat Counter (A. Natow and J. Heslin, New York: Simon & Schuster, 1989)

The T-Factor (J. Pope-Cordle and M. Kabahn, New York: W.W. Norton, 1991)

CARBOHYDRATE COUNTING

Bowes and Church's Food Values of Portions Commonly Used, 15th ed. (Joan Pennington, Philadelphia: J.B. Lippincott, 1989)

Calories and Carbohydrates (Barbara Kraus, New York: New American Library, 1988)

The Complete Book of Food Counts (Corinne T. Netzer, New York: Bantam/Doubleday Dell, 1988)

The Complete Calorie and Carbohydrate Counter for Dining Out (Kathryn Ernst, New York: Simon & Schuster, 1987)

Food Choice Lists

MILK LIST

Best Choices:

Nonfat or low-fat

Be Sure:

You take calcium supplements if you use less than 2 cups per day for adults, 3–4 cups per day for children.

NONFAT SELECTIONS

One choice provides:

Calories: 80	Carb: 12 grams
Protein: 8 grams	Fat: 0 gram

ITEM	PORTION
Nonfat milk (skim)	1 cup
Low-fat milk (½%)	1 cup
Nonfat yogurt made with NutraSweet, e.g., Yoplait Light, Weight Watchers Ultimate 90, Colombo Slender Spoonfuls Dannon Light	6–8 oz

Regular fruited yogurt	
Fat Free Colombo	3 oz
Lactaid milk (skim)	1 cup
Powdered, nonfat milk	
(before adding liquid)	⅓ cup
Canned, evaporated skim milk	½ cup
Sugar-free hot cocoa mix plus 6 oz	
of water*	1 cup

*Most cocoa mixes do not provide the same amount of calcium as one cup of milk. Compare labels on mixes for the amount of calcium that the product contains. An example of a product that meets these calcium requirements is Alba sugar-free, hot cocoa mix.

LOW-FAT SELECTIONS
One choice provides:

Calories: 107	Carb: 12 grams
Protein: 8 grams	Fat: 3 grams

ITEM	PORTION
Low-fat milk (1%)	1 cup
Yogurt, plain, unflavored	1 cup
Regular fruited yogurt	
Yoplait Lowfat	½ cup
Dannon Lowfat	3 oz
Lactaid milk (1%)	1 cup

MEDIUM- AND HIGH-FAT

The following milk items should be used sparingly due to their high saturated fat and cholesterol content.

One choice provides:

Calories: 125–150	Carb: 12 grams
Protein: 8 grams	Fat: 5–8 grams

ITEM	PORTION
Low-fat milk (2%)	1 cup
Whole milk	1 cup

Vegetable List

Best Choices:

Fresh or raw vegetables: dark green, leafy, or orange

Be Sure:

To choose at least 2 vegetables each day.

We Encourage:

Steaming with a minimum amount of water.

One choice provides:

Calories: 28	Carb: 5 grams
Protein: 2 grams	Fat: 0 gram

ITEM	PORTION
Artichoke	one half
Asparagus	1 cup
Bamboo shoots	½ cup
Bean sprouts	½ cup
Beets	½ cup
Beet greens	1 cup
Broccoli	½ cup
Brussels sprouts	½ cup
Cabbage	1 cup
Carrots	½ cup
Cauliflower	1 cup
Celery	1 cup
Collard greens	1 cup
Eggplant	½ cup
Fennel leaf	1 cup
Green beans	1 cup
Green pepper	1 cup
Kale	½ cup
Kohlrabi	½ cup
Leeks	½ cup
Mushrooms, fresh	1 cup
Mustard greens, cooked	1 cup
Okra	½ cup

Onion	½ cup
Pea pods, Chinese (snow peas)	½ cup
Radishes	1 cup
Red pepper	1 cup
Rutabagas	½ cup
*Sauerkraut	½ cup
Spinach, cooked	½ cup
Squash	
summer	1 cup
zucchini	1 cup
Swiss chard	1 cup
Tomato (ripe)	1 medium
*Tomato juice	½ cup
Tomato paste	1½ tbsp
*Tomato sauce, canned	⅓ cup
Turnips	½ cup
Vegetables, mixed	¼ cup
*V-8 juice	½ cup
Wax beans	1 cup
Water chestnuts	5 whole

Because of their low carbohydrate and calorie content, the following RAW vegetables may be used liberally.

Alfalfa sprouts
Chicory
Chinese cabbage
Cucumber
Endive
Escarole
Lettuce
Parsley
*Pickles (unsweetened)
Pimento
Spinach
Watercress

*These vegetables are high in sodium (salt). Low-sodium vegetables, juices, and sauces should be purchased if you are following a sodium-restricted diet. Fresh and frozen vegetables are lower in sodium than canned vegetables, unless the canned product states "low sodium."

FRUIT LIST

Best Choices:

Fresh whole fruit

Be Sure:

To choose fresh, frozen, or canned fruit packed in its own juice or water with no added sugar.

One choice provides:

Calories: 60	Carb: 15 grams
Protein: 0 gram	Fat: 0 gram

ITEM	PORTION
Apple, 2-inch diameter	1 small
Apple, dried	¼ cup
Applesauce	½ cup
Apricots	
fresh	4 medium
canned	4 halves
dried	7 halves
Banana, 9-inch length, peeled	½
Banana flakes or chips	3 tbsp
Blackberries	¾ cup
Blueberries	¾ cup
Boysenberries	1 cup
Canned fruit, unless otherwise stated	½ cup
Cantaloupe, 5-inch diameter	
sectioned	⅓ melon
cubed	1 cup
Casaba, 7-inch diameter	
sectioned	⅙ melon
cubed	1⅓ cup
Cherries, sweet fresh	12
Dates	3
Figs	2 small
Granadilla (passion fruit)	4
Grapefruit, 4-inch diameter	½
Grapes	15 small

Guava	1½ small
Honeydew melon, 6½-inch diameter	
sectioned	⅛ melon
cubed	1 cup
Kiwi (3 oz)	1 large
Kumquat	5 medium
Lemon	1 large
Loquats, fresh	12
Lychees, fresh or dried	10
Mango	½ small
sliced	½ cup
Nectarine, 2½-inch diameter	1
Orange, 3-inch diameter	1
Papaya, 3½-inch diameter	
sectioned	½
cubed	1 cup
Peach, 2½-inch diameter	1
Pear	1 small
Persimmon	
native	2
Japanese, 2½-inch diameter	½
Pineapple	
fresh, diced	¾ cup
canned	⅓ cup
Plantain, cooked	⅓ cup
Plum, 2-inch diameter	2
Pomegranate, 3½-inch diameter	½
Prunes, dried, medium	3
Raisins	2 tbsp
Raspberries	1 cup
Rhubarb, fresh, diced	3 cups
Strawberries	1⅓ cups
Tangerine, 2½-inch diameter	2
Watermelon, diced	1¼ cups

Fruit Juice

ITEM	PORTION
Apple juice, unsweetened	4 oz
Cranapple, low-calorie	12 oz

Cranberry, low-calorie	10 oz
Grape juice, unsweetened	4 oz
Grapefruit juice, unsweetened	5 oz
Lemon juice, unsweetened	6 oz
Orange juice, unsweetened	4 oz
Pineapple juice, unsweetened	4 oz
Prune juice, unsweetened	3 oz
Twister, Light (with NutraSweet)	8 oz
Twister regular	4 oz

BREAD/STARCH LIST

Best Choices:

Whole-grain breads and cereals, dried beans and peas.
(In general, one bread choice equals 1 oz of bread.)

BREADS

One choice provides:

Calories: 80	Carb: 15 grams
Protein: 3 grams	Fat: trace

ITEM	PORTION
White, whole-wheat, rye, etc.	1 slice
Raisin	1 slice
Italian and French	1 slice
Reduced calorie	
(1 slice equals 40 calories)	2 slices
Syrian	
pocket, 6-inch diameter	½ pocket
diet size	1 pocket
Bagel	½ medium
English muffin	½ medium
Rolls	
bulkie	½ small
dinner, plain	1 small
frankfurter	½ medium
hamburger	½ medium
Bread crumbs	3 tbsp

BREAKFAST ITEMS

	SERVING	EXCHANGES
NutriGrain bar with fruit	1	1 bread + ½ fruit
Pepperidge Farms Whole-some Choice Muffins (corn, apple, raisin bran, or blueberry)	1	1 bread + 1 fruit
Healthy Choice Blueberry Muffin	1	1 bread + 1½ fruit + 1 fat

CEREALS

ITEM	PORTION
Cooked cereals	½ cup
Bran	
†All Bran with Extra Fiber	1 cup
†All Bran	⅓ cup
†100% Bran	⅔ cup
†40% Bran Flakes	½ cup
†Bran Chex	½ cup
Multibran Chex	⅓ cup
†Fiber One	⅔ cup
Cheerios	1 cup
Common Sense Oat Bran	½ cup
Corn, Rice Chex	⅔ cup
Cornflakes	¾ cup
Crispix	½ cup
Fortified Oat Flakes	½ cup
Frosted Flakes	⅓ cup
Granola: Kellogg's lowfat	⅛ cup
Grapenuts	3 tbsp
†Grapenut Flakes	⅔ cup
Just Right (with fiber nuggets)	½ cup
Kenmei Rice Bran	½ cup
Kix	1 cup
NutriGrain	½ cup
Product 19	½ cup
Puffed Rice, Wheat	1½ cups
Rice Krispies	¾ cup
†Shredded Wheat biscuit	1
spoon size	½ cup

†Shredded Wheat 'n' Bran	½ cup
Special K	¾ cup
Team	⅔ cup
Total	¾ cup
Trix	½ cup
†Wheat Chex	½ cup
†Wheaties	⅔ cup
Other cold cereals	⅔ cup

†Cereals high in fiber.

STARCHY VEGETABLES

ITEM	PORTION
Corn	½ cup
Corn on the cob	
5 × 1¾-inch length	1
Lima beans	½ cup
Parsnips	½ cup
Peas, green, canned, or frozen	⅔ cup
Plantain, cooked	⅓ cup
Potato, white	
mashed	½ cup
baked	½ medium or 1 small (3 oz)
Sweet potato	
mashed	⅓ cup
baked	½ medium (2 oz)
Pumpkin	¾ cup
Winter squash, acorn, or butternut	¾ cup

PASTA
(cooked)

Macaroni, noodles, spaghetti	½ cup

LEGUMES

Beans, peas, lentils	
(dried and cooked)	⅓ cup
Baked beans, canned, no pork	
(vegetarian style)	⅓ cup

GRAINS

Barley, cooked	¼ cup
Bulgur, cooked	⅓ cup
Cornmeal	2½ tbsp
Cornstarch	2 tbsp
Flour	3 tbsp
Kasha, cooked	⅓ cup
Rice, cooked	⅓ cup
Wheat germ	¼ cup = 1 bread + 1 lean meat

CRACKERS/COOKIES EQUAL TO ONE BREAD CHOICE

Best Choices:

Lower sodium products, e.g., saltines with unsalted tops

ITEM	PORTION
AK-mak, regular and sesame	4 crackers
Animal crackers	8
Crokine puffed crispbread	4
Finn Crisp	4
Gingersnaps	3
Graham crackers 2½-inch squares	3
Granola bar lowfat Nature Valley, Quaker	½ bar
Health Valley Cookies	3
Krispen: crispbread	4
Matzoh or matzoh with bran	1 (¾ oz)
Manischewitz whole-wheat matzoh crackers	7
Melba toast rectangles	5
Melba toast rounds	10
Norwegian flatbread such as Kavli thin	3
thick	2
Pepperidge Farm Wholesome Choice Oatmeal Raisin Cookies	2 = 1 bread + ½ fruit
Popcorn, popped, no fat added	3 cups
Orville Redenbacher's SmartPop	4 cups

Potato chips, fatfree
    Childers, Michael Season's   15
*Pretzel   ¾ oz
*Mr. Phipps pretzel chips   12
Rice cakes, popcorn cakes   2
    Mini rice cakes   8
Ry-Krisp, triple crackers   3
Ryvita: crisp breads   4
*Saltines   6
Snackwells fatfree wheat crackers   6
    cheddar crackers   24
Social Teas   4
Stella d'Oro Almond Toast   1½
Stella d'Oro Egg Biscuit   2
Stoned Wheat Thins   2½
Tortilla, Guiltless Gourmet,
    no oil tortilla chip   8
Triscuit, reduced fat   5
Uneedas   4
Wasa Lite or Golden Rye or
    Hearty Ry-Krisp Bread   2
Zwieback   3

*High in sodium.

CRACKERS FOR OCCASIONAL USE

(equal to one bread plus one fat choice)

ITEM	PORTION
Arrowroot	4
Bordeaux Cookies, Pepperidge Farm	3
*Butter crackers	
rounds	7
rectangular	6
*Cheez-its	27
*Cheez Nips	20
reduced fat	22 = 1 bread + ½ fat
*Club or Townhouse Crackers	6
*Combos	1 oz
*Escort Crackers	5

Frookies	2
*Goldfish, Pepperidge Farm	36
Granola bar, plain, raisin, or peanut butter	1
Lorna Doones	3
*Meal Mates	5
Mr. Phipps Tater Crisps (original, BBQ, or Sour Cream 'n Onion)	16 = 1 bread + ½ fat
Nabisco lowfat garden crisps	9 = 1 bread + ½ fat
*Oyster crackers	24
*Peanut Butter Sandwich Crackers	3
Popcorn: Orville Redenbacher's Light	4 cups
*Ritz	7
*Sea Rounds	2
*Sociables	9
Stella d'Oro Sesame Breadsticks	2
Stella d'Oro Breakfast Treats	1
Stella d'Oro Golden Bar	1
Stella d'Oro Lady Stella Assortment	3
*Sunshine Hi Ho's	6
Teddy Grahams	15
*Tidbits	21
Triscuits	5
Vanilla Wafers	6
Wasa Fiber Plus Crisp Bread	4
Wasa Sesame or Breakfast Crisp Bread	2
*Waverly Wafers	6
*Wheat Thins	12
reduced fat	13 = 1 bread + ½ fat

* High in Sodium.

MEAT LIST

Best Choices:

Nonfat or low-fat selections

Be Sure:

To trim off visible fat. To bake, broil, or steam selections with no added fat. To weigh your portion after cooking.

We Encourage:

Portions to be the accompaniment rather than the main course.

NONFAT SELECTIONS
One choice provides:

Calories: 40–45	Carb: 0 gram
Protein: 7 grams	Fat: 0 gram

ITEM	PORTION
Nonfat cheese products:	
*Alpine Lace Free 'n Lean Cheese	1 oz
*Hood Free cottage cheese	¼ cup
*Calabro 100% skim ricotta	1 oz
*Kraft Free Singles	1 oz

LOW-FAT SELECTIONS
One choice provides:

Calories: 55	Carb: 0 gram
Protein: 7 grams	Fat: 3 grams

ITEM	PORTION
Cheese:	
Cottage, 1% fat, Dragone Lite Ricotta	¼ cup
Axelrod's nonfat, sugar-free with pineapple	½ cup = 2 lean meat + ½ fruit
*Lite-Line cheese, *Nuform cheese, Weight Watchers cheese, Laughing Cow, Smartbeat Singles, Light n' Lively Free	1 oz
Cooked dried beans	½ cup = 1 meat + 1 bread
Egg substitute with less than 55 calories per ¼ cup	½ cup
Egg whites	3
Fish and seafood:	
Fresh or frozen	1 oz

Canned:

Herring, uncreamed or *smoked	1 oz
Imitation crab	1 oz
Sardines, drained	3
Water-packed clams, oysters, scallops, **shrimp	1 oz
Water-packed salmon, tuna, crab, **lobster	¼ cup
Healthy Choice 96% fat-free ground beef	1 oz
Hot dogs 97% fat-free	1 (2 oz) = 2 lean meats
*Luncheon meat, 95% fat-free, turkey ham	1 oz
Poultry: chicken, turkey, or Cornish hen, without skin	1 oz
Ground chicken, turkey meat	1 oz
*Canadian bacon	1 oz
Tofu	3 oz
Turkey sausage	1 oz

* High in sodium.
** People trying to reduce dietary cholesterol may need to limit these. For additional information, ask your dietitian.

MEDIUM-FAT SELECTIONS

One choice provides:

Calories: 75	Carb: 0 gram
Protein: 7 grams	Fat: 5 grams

ITEM	PORTION
Veal, except for breast	1 oz
Pork, except for deviled ham, ground pork, and spare ribs	1 oz
Beef, chipped, chuck, flank steak; hamburger with 15% fat, rib eye, rump, sirloin, tenderloin top and bottom round	1 oz
Lamb, except for breast	1 oz

Cheese:

    Part-skim mozzarella, part-skim
    ricotta, farmer, Neufchatel,
    Velveeta light, Tasty-Lo sharp
    cheddar cheese spread, Jarlsberg
    Light, Dormans Slim Jack
    reduced-fat Monterey, Cracker
    Barrel Light, Cabot Light
    Vitalait, Kraft Light   1 oz
  *Parmesan, *Romano   3 tbsp
***Egg   1
    Egg substitute with 50–80 calories
      per ¼ cup   ¼ cup
  *Luncheon meat, 86% fat-free
      turkey bologna, turkey salami   1 oz
    Turkey bacon   2 slices
    Peanut butter   1 tbsp = 1 meat + 1 fat
    Turkey franks   1 (1.6 oz) = 1½ med.
                             meat

* High in sodium.
*** Eggs are high in cholesterol. Limit consumption to 3–4 per week.

Be Sure:

That the high-fat meat choices listed below are used sparingly, due to the high saturated fat and cholesterol content.

HIGH-FAT SELECTIONS

One choice provides:

Calories: 100	Carb: 0 gram
Protein: 7 grams	Fat: 8 grams

ITEM	PORTION
Beef:	

brisket, club and rib steak,
    *corned beef, regular hamburger
    with 20% fat, rib roast, short ribs
	1 oz

Lamb: breast	1 oz

Pork:
  *deviled ham, ground pork, spare
  ribs, *sausage (patty or link)   1 oz
Veal: breast   1 oz
Poultry:
  capon, duck, goose   1 oz
Regular cheese:
  *blue, Brie, cheddar, Colby, *feta,
  Monterey Jack, Muenster,
  provolone, Swiss,
  *pasteurized process   1 oz
*Luncheon meats:
  bologna, bratwurst,
  braunschweiger, knockwurst,
  liverwurst, pastrami, Polish
  sausage, salami   1 oz
Organ meats:
  liver, heart, kidney   1 oz
Fried fish   1 oz

* High in sodium.

FAT LIST

Best Choices:

More unsaturated selections

Be Sure:

When using low-calorie version of fat choices, to use amounts equal to
45 calories for one serving.

One choice provides:	
Calories: 45	Carb: 0 gram
Protein: 0 gram	Fat: 5 grams

MORE UNSATURATED

ITEM	PORTION
Avocado, 4-inch diameter	1/8
D-Zerta, whipped topping	5 tbsp

Margarine, soft tub or *stick	1 tsp
Reduced calories: Promise Ultra, Promise Extralite, Mazola Extralite, Fleischmann's Extralite, Promise Light, Latta	1 tbsp
**Mayonnaise	1 tsp
Reduced calories	1 tbsp
Nondairy creamer, liquid	2 tbsp
Nondairy creamer, lite, liquid	5 tbsp
Nuts	
Almonds	6 whole
Brazil	2 medium
Cashews	5–8 whole
Filberts (hazelnuts)	5 whole
Macadamia	3 whole
Peanuts	
Spanish	20 whole
Virginia	10 whole
Pecans	2 whole
Pignolia (pine nuts)	1 tbsp
Pistachio	12 whole
Walnuts	2 whole
Other	1 tbsp
Oils:	
Corn, cottonseed, safflower, soy, sunflower, olive, peanut (monounsaturated)	1 tsp
Olives:	
green	5 small
black	2 large
Salad dressings:	
**French, Italian	1 tbsp
Mayonnaise type	2 tsp
*Seeds (without shells)	
sesame, sunflower	1 tbsp
pumpkin	2 tsp

* High in sodium.
** Can be used in a cholesterol-reducing diet if made with corn, cottonseed, safflower, soy, or sunflower oil as the first ingredient.

MORE SATURATED

ITEM	PORTION
Bacon, crisp	1 strip
Butter	1 tsp
Chitterlings	½ oz
Coconut, shredded	2 tbsp
Coffee whitener, liquid	2 tbsp
Coffee whitener, powder	4 tbsp
Cool Whip	3 tbsp
Cream	
Half and half	2 tbsp
Heavy	1 tbsp
Light	1½ tbsp
Sour	2 tbsp
Hood Light	4 tbsp
Whipped, fluid	1 tbsp
Whipped, pressurized topping	⅓ cup
Cream cheese: Philadelphia Light	1 tbsp
Whipped	2 tbsp
Lard	1 tsp
Margarine, stick	
(oil not listed as first ingredient)	1 tsp
Oils:	
palm, coconut	1 tsp
Salad dressings:	
(oil not listed as first ingredient)	
*French, Italian	1 tbsp
Seven Seas Light Italian	
with Olive Oil	2 tbsp
Mayonnaise type	2 tsp
Salt pork	¼ oz

*High in sodium.

FAT SUBSTITUTES AND CONDIMENTS FOR LOW-FAT DIETS

Many fat-free substitutes contain 1 or more types of sugar. Although the amount of sweetener is small, it is important to use no more than *1 teaspoon* of the jam or no more than *20 calories* of a condiment.

One choice provides:

A free exchange

ITEM	PORTION
Sour cream	
Light 'n Lively Free	2 tbsp
Margarine and mayonnaise	
Cain's Fat-Free Mayonnaise	1 tbsp
Kraft Fat-Free Mayonnaise	1 tbsp
Kraft Miracle Whip Free	1 tbsp
Butter Buds	½ tsp
Molly McButter	½ tsp
Cream cheese	
Philadelphia Free	2 tbsp
Gravy	
Pepperidge Farm 98% Fat-Free Gravies	2 tbsp
Salad dressings	
Kraft Free	
Italian	1 tbsp
Ranch	1 tbsp
Catalina	1 tbsp
Blue Cheese	1 tbsp
Good Seasons Free	
Zesty Herb	1 tbsp
Italian	1 tbsp
Creamy Italian	1 tbsp
Seven Seas Free	
Italian	1 tbsp
Red Wine Vinegar	1 tbsp
Wishbone Healthy Sensation	
Chunky Blue Cheese	1 tbsp
Honey Dijon	1 tbsp
Wishbone Lite	
Italian	1 tbsp
Pritikin	
Garlic & Herb	1 tbsp
Jams	
Smuckers Simply Fruit	1 tsp
Smuckers Low-Sugar Spread	1 tsp
Polaner All Fruit	1 tsp
Polaner Lite	1 tsp

MISCELLANEOUS LIST

Many foods are made up of several food groups. These mixed foods can be incorporated into your meal plan by substituting them for choices from more than one food group.

*Canned Soup

ITEM	PORTION	FOOD CHOICE
Rice or noodle with broth prepared with water	8 oz	½ bread, ½ fat
Campbell's Healthy Request Chowder	8 oz	1 bread
Chunky style, ready to serve	8 oz	1 bread, 1 meat, 1 vegetable
Cream soup Made with water	8 oz	½ bread, 1½ fat
Made with 1% low-fat milk	8 oz	½ bread, ½ milk, 1½ fat
Clam chowder, New England style, prepared with 1% low-fat milk	8 oz	½ bread, 1 milk, 1 fat
Lentil with ham, ready to serve	8 oz	1 bread, 1 meat, 1 vegetable
Minestrone, ready to serve	8 oz	1 bread, 1 vegetable
Split pea with ham, ready to serve	8 oz	2 bread, 1½ meat
Tomato, made with water	8 oz	1 bread

* High in sodium unless specially prepared without salt.

Prepared Foods

ITEM	PORTION	FOOD CHOICE
Angel food cake	⅙ Betty Crocker cake mix	1 bread
Biscuit	2-inch diameter (1 oz)	1 bread + 1 fat
Cornbread	2 x 2 x 1 inch	1 bread + 1 fat
Muffin, bran or corn	2-inch diameter (1½ oz)	1½ bread + 1 fat
Granola	¼ cup	1 bread + 1 fat
Pancake	4-inch diameter	2 = 1 bread + 1 fat
Waffle	4-inch diameter	1 bread + 1 fat
Eggowaffle Special K	4-inch diameter	1 bread
Taco shells	2	1 bread + 1 fat
Taco	1	2 meat, 1 bread, 1 fat
Tortilla		
corn	6-inch diameter	2 = 1 bread + 1 fat
flour	7-inch diameter	1 bread + 1 fat
*Plain cheese pizza	⅛ of 14-inch diameter	1 bread, 1 meat, 1 vegetable, 1 fat
Lasagna, homemade	2½ x 2½ x 1¾ inch	1 bread, 3 meat, 2 vegetable, 1 fat
*Ravioli, canned	1 cup	1 bread, 1 meat, 1 vegetable
Beef stew, homemade	1 cup	3 meat, 1 bread, 1 vegetable
Chili with meat and beans, homemade	1 cup	3 meat, 2 bread
*Spaghetti with meat, canned	1 cup	1½ bread, 1 vegetable, 1 meat, 1 fat

| Popcorn, microwave, light | 3 cups | 1 bread + 1 fat |

* High sodium unless specially prepared without salt.

Desserts/Sweets

ITEM	PORTION	FOOD CHOICE
Frozen iced milk	½ cup	1 bread + 1 fat
Pudding, sugar-free, made with skim or 1% low-fat milk	½ cup	½ milk + ½ bread
Chunks O'Fruit All Fruit fruit bar	1 bar	1 fruit
Pancake syrup		
Regular	1 tbsp	1 bread
Lite	2 tbsp	1 bread
Sugar-Free	2 tbsp	free
Sugar	1 tbsp	1 bread
Honey	1 tbsp	1 bread
Regular jelly	1 tbsp	1 bread
All-fruit	1 tbsp	1 bread
Low-sugar jelly	1 tbsp	1 bread

Frozen Treats

Best Choice:

Nonfat, sugar-free products are recommended as the best choice because of their low-sugar, low-fat content.

ITEM	PORTION	FOOD CHOICE
Fudgesicle Sugar-Free Popsicle	1 bar	free
Sugar-Free Fudgesicle	1 bar	½ bread
Weight Watchers Chocolate Mousse Bars	1 bar	½ bread
Weight Watchers Orange Vanilla Treat	1 bar	½ bread
Hendries Fudge Stix	1 bar	½ bread

ITEM	PORTION	FOOD CHOICE
SOFT SERVE, NONFAT, SUGAR-FREE		
Freshens, Honey Hill Farms, I Can't Believe It's Yogurt, TCBY, Baskin-Robbins sugar-free ice cream, Simple Pleasures Light frozen dairy dessert	½ cup	1 bread
SOFT SERVE		
Columbo low-fat, Dannon Light nonfat, frozen yogurt, Everything Yogurt nonfat and low-fat, Honey Hill Farms nonfat, I Can't Believe It's Yogurt nonfat	½ cup	1 bread
Columbo nonfat, Dairy Queen nonfat vanilla, Dannon low-fat, Freshens low-fat and nonfat, McDonald's, TCBY nonfat	½ cup	1½ bread

Foods for Occasional Use

Be Sure:

Because of the high-fat and/or calorie content of the following foods, use only occasionally, i.e., not more than once or twice per week. Count the fat exchanges in your meal plan.

ITEM	PORTION	FOOD CHOICE
Croissant	4 x 4 x 1¾ inch	2 bread + 2 fats
Ice cream	½ cup	1 bread + 2 fats

Potatoes, french fries, 2 to 3½-inch length	10	1 bread + 2 fats
Potato or corn chips	15	1 bread + 2 fats
Stuffing mix, cooked	⅓ cup	1 bread + 2 fats
Potato or macaroni salad made with regular mayonnaise	½ cup	1 bread + 2 fats
Hot dog	1	1 high-fat meat + 1 fat

Free Foods

The following foods contain very few calories and may be used freely in your meal plan. Items marked with an asterisk (*) should not be used, however, if you are on a salt- (sodium) restricted diet.

GENERAL

*Bouillon cubes
Bran, unprocessed (1 tbsp)
*Broth (clear)
Calorie-free soft drinks
*Catsup (1 tbsp daily—calculated as part of the total daily calories)
Coffee
*Consommé
Cranberries (unsweetened)
Decaffeinated coffee
Extracts (see list opposite)
Herbs (see list opposite)
Horseradish
Lime juice
Lemon/lime rind
*Mustard (prepared)
Noncaloric sugar substitute

Orange rind
*Pickles (unsweetened)
Postum (limited to 3 cups daily unless calculated as part of the total daily calories)
Rennet tablets
Seasonings and condiments (see list opposite)
*Soy sauce
Spices (see list opposite)
*Steak sauce
Tabasco sauce
Taco sauce
Tea
Vinegar (cider, white, apple, wine)
Yeast (dry or cake)

SPICES, HERBS, AND EXTRACTS

Allspice	Fennel
Almond extract	Garlic
Anise extract	Ginger
Baking powder	Lemon extract
*Baking soda	Mace
Basil	Maple extract
Bay leaf	Mint
Black cherry extract	Mustard (dry)
*Bouillon cube	Nutmeg
Butter flavoring	Onion (1 tbsp)
*Butter salt	Orange extract
Caraway seeds	Oregano
Cardamom	Paprika
*Celery salt (seeds, leaves)	Parsley
Chives	Pepper
Chocolate extract	Peppermint extract
Cilantro (Mexican coriander)	Pimento
Cinnamon	Poppy seed
Cloves	Poultry seasonings
Cream of tartar	Saffron
Cumin	Sage
Curry	*Salt
Dill	Savory

Acknowledgments

Developing a book such as this is truly a monumental team effort requiring the assistance of many different types of experts. As we worked on this book and had to decide what exactly to put down in black and white about how to treat a particular aspect of diabetes, we came to appreciate how much of medicine is an imprecise art, as well as a precise science.

We want to thank all the members of the Joslin staff—past and present—who helped develop, review, and debate the content of this book. This includes the entire current membership of the Joslin Education Committee who gave us their thoughts and expertise in reviewing various sections of the book: Laurinda Poirier, R.N., M.P.H.; Barbara Anderson, Ph.D., C.D.E.; Cynthia Pasquarello, R.N., C.D.E.; Melinda Maryniuk, R.D., C.D.E.; Joy Kistler, M.S., C.D.E.

Others involved in reviewing specific chapters included Sue Ghiloni, R.N., C.D.E.; John Hare, M.D.; Florence Brown, M.D.; Julie Goodwin, P.A.-C, C.D.E.; Carol Jensen, R.N.; Annette Alderman, R.N., C.D.E.; Jerry Cavallerano, O.D., Ph.D.; and Beverly Halford, R.D., C.D.E. Donna Richardson, R.N., C.D.E., was instrumental in developing the first and second drafts of this work, as was Chris Aho, who worked diligently to help us all put our thoughts together. When it came time to finally put this book to bed, Ray Moloney, Julie Rafferty, and Tom McCullough worked tirelessly proofing and copyediting to see that we met deadlines and that our information was clear. Brenetta Ingram provided important secretarial support to our efforts.

To all of the above people, we give our thanks in enabling us to bring this book to people with diabetes, to help you live well with this disease.

Richard S. Beaser, M.D.
Joan V. C. Hill, R.D., C.D.E.

Index